CHRIS AND ERIC MARTINEZ

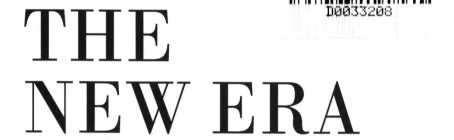

THE
NEW ERA
OF FITNESS

8 Proven Habits to Double Your Strength, Sexiness, Energy,
Health, and Live a Well-Balanced Dynamic Lifestyle

First Edition 2016

Printed in the United States of America

Published by:
Dynamic Duo Training
2045 S State College Blvd
Anaheim, CA 92806
www.DynamicDuoTraining.com

For more information about Eric and Chris Martinez or to book them for your next event, speaking engagement, podcast or media interview please visit: www. DynamicDuoTraining.com

Dedication/Acknowledgements

This book is dedicated to the following people that have blessed our lives and helped us unlock our true potential:

Our courageous mother, Maria Martinez, and awesome older brother, Mike, who we look up to so much.

Chris's beautiful and supportive girlfriend, Lissette.

Our friends back home in Santa Rosa and our friends here in Orange County who have supported us through thick and thin.

Our DDT community and clients, who we learn so much from every day.

Our mentors and coaches for always pushing us and leading by example.

Our business partner Rory Carruthers, who contributed so much to make this book a reality.

Our editor, Carly Carruthers, who provided so much more than checking grammar and punctuation.

Everyone who has enriched our life, you know who you are. Thank you!

Table of Contents

Preface

The Night Everything Changed

It's 4 a.m. in the morning, 3 days before Christmas, you and your identical twin are 18 years old, you're seniors in high school, and everything in your life is going so well; life couldn't be better. A priest and a police officer knock on your door, you both run into your older brother's and parents' rooms to see if they're all there... Your father is not there.

Your heart sinks to the floor, and you ask, "Where's my dad?"

The priest and police officer sit the family down and tell us that our father has been killed in a car accident.

We can't process it, we can't breathe, we are cold and have chills running down our spines, and our vision is blurry...the only thing we can hear is our mother screaming and crying, "Nooooooo!"

Our life has just been turned upside down as fast as you can snap your fingers.

We begin to realize that our 18 years of happiness was just crushed, and for what reason? Nobody will ever know. That so called light of happiness just got a dark cloud over it, and we realized our family will never be the same again.

We entered hell at the age of 18 and knew we had a long road ahead of us to get back. We had the picture perfect life, and now it was all gone and taken from us.

1

We knew that our ultimate provider, our leader, our role model to mold us into men, our father wasn't there to guide us in life anymore. We knew a piece of our mother went with him that night, and she would never be the same again. We knew our older brother would have to take on that father figure role at such a young age and be robbed of anything else he planned on doing.

Three months after our father passed away, we found out our closest grandmother, our mom's mother, was diagnosed with cancer. Our grandmother battled her cancer for a few months and then passed away. Three years later, our grandma and grandpa on our dad's side passed away as well. Another ton of bricks hit us, especially our mother, she was so lost. We could not understand why this was happening to our family.

Our First Mentor

Growing up, we lived a very structured life with school, sports, church, and family time. Our father was a Correctional Officer at San Quentin State Prison before he passed away, so you can imagine he was pretty strict and made sure we had daily structure. He once told us, "Nothing in life will ever be given to you, you have to work for everything you want and if it's too easy, then find something bigger that challenges you." Everything he had taught us up to that point would have to be practiced in the real world on our own. Trial and error, as society likes to call it.

Our father had a relentless mindset; he was the ultimate provider for our family and one hell of a role model to us. We get our personality and wild side from our mom, which is a great balance. We watched our father's work ethic each and every day, and that rubbed off on us. When he passed away, we had our dark times; however, we found a way out because we were relentless as well.

We knew we were always in the fight and to never ever quit. We prevailed after many years of battling.

After his death, we made a promise to ourselves that we would be there by our mother's side for however long it took us to graduate college at the local Sonoma State University.

We would sacrifice not going away to college, we would sacrifice not getting the college experience by living on campus, we would sacrifice not being able to take spring breaks to exotic destinations like normal college students do, and we would work to help pay tuition and bills at home.

This wasn't the way it was supposed to go down for us. But we survived the curveball, the tragedy that occurred, and we manned up and did what we had to do to get through it. We developed a relentless mindset and a form of mental toughness that we never knew we had inside of us.

The Power of Fitness - Our Way Back

We wrote this book because over the past decade, fitness saved our lives. Going into the gym and taking our anger out on the iron was our only outlet. It helped us focus on overall health and taught us how to manage our stress better. It gave us structure and something to look forward to each day while we constantly progressed and challenged ourselves.

It helped mold us into the men that we are today, helped us overcome adversity, helped us create Dynamic Duo Training, and created this insatiable hunger to never settle for less and to always keep our feet on the gas pedal no matter what life has in store for us.

We realized that this past decade we made a ton of mistakes within fitness and our personal life, but it's a blessing in disguise because if we didn't make so many mistakes, we couldn't have ever written this book to help you. The challenges we experienced and the lessons we learned can help you on your journey to improved fitness and health.

This book is not a bullshit fad or "get fit quick" kind of book; it's intended to enhance your fitness journey through exercise, nutrition, lifestyle, and mindset, and to accelerate your results.

This book is going to make you realize that the New Era of Fitness is here, whether you like it or not, and it's up to YOU to adapt to it and benefit from it.

Introduction

Everything in Life Evolves, Why Not Fitness?

The question should also be, why not now? The New Era of Fitness should be flexible, enjoyable, realistic, and challenging. It should be constantly changing to optimize your results in all areas of your life, such as: mentality, social life, work, health, wealth, love, and happiness. Fitness shouldn't be looked at under a microscope, nor as black and white through just exercise and nutrition; it should, and needs, to be looked at as constant change and optimization through all aspects of life.

We could write an entire book on how much dogma, misleading information, and unethical practices we have seen and heard from current and past clients and our colleagues. The fitness industry has its pros and cons, just like any other industry. There are good people trying to actually help others and make change, then there are those who are shady, trying to make a quick buck, and don't give a shit. We are firm believers in what goes around, comes around. You can only fake something for so long before you are exposed and finished with your name and business for good.

Our Core Values

Before we got into coaching, we hired our first coach Dr. Layne Norton. He taught us everything we know and inspired us to start our own business. We hope you'll take the time to learn more about

5

Dr. Layne Norton and his philosophy/teachings at Biolayne.com. From there on, we continued to hire more and more mentors to gain more knowledge and add more tools to our arsenal. Within the pages of New Era of Fitness, you'll learn about all of our mentors and their teachings. We remember Layne telling us, "Integrity is everything. If you treat your customer's right, they will love you and you will thrive." This really resonated with us and our Core Values, which are:

- Integrity
- Legacy
- Family
- Relationships
- Success

Once we got the opportunity to coach a few clients, everything took off for us. That is why we are so successful to this day with our business Dynamic Duo Training. We were never afraid to be ourselves, take risks, ask for help, reach out to bigger names, treat people right, put out honest and quality content, and be open to change and learn more.

Evolution is Key

Many people in all industries today do not want to embrace change. We cannot understand why, as we are in the most exciting time to live and evolve as a society. Perhaps people are just arrogant or close minded and feel their way is the best and nothing else matters. We have seen a lot of this in the fitness industry; people do not like to be wrong or they feel like they know the answer to everything just to satisfy their own egos. It truly is a shame because we are all a constant work in progress and should be students to everything to keep expanding our knowledge. Our business mentor Tai Lopez, an investor, speaker, author and entrepreneur at www. tailopez.com, once told us, "A mind full of conclusions has no room for expansion."

We wrote this book because we are huge advocates of change, and we love to lead by example. We are educators and coaches who are always looking for ways to evolve, enhance our client's mental and physical state, leverage our business, and constantly learn from others. We want others to be the best versions of themselves each and every day, and we want to see others succeed. We have been through a ton of adversity and failed along our journey, but most importantly, we have learned from our mistakes, have never made any excuses, and have become quite successful along the way. We know everyone has their own battles in life. Life itself is a constant grind and roller coaster, but anything is possible if you put in the work and keep climbing up that mountain, inch by inch. Many people want to take the elevator to success, when you should be taking the stairs.

A Dynamic Lifestyle

Nothing great or worth-while happens overnight; neither should one trying to change their life and overall health. We have come up with 8 proven strategies to double your strength, sexiness, energy, health, and how to live a well-balanced Dynamic Lifestyle. These are eight areas of focus, health, and continual improvement.

1. **Now is the time to become Dynamic!** Everyone thinks there is a perfect time to start something or make a change. New Year's resolutions are once per year and are complete bullshit. If you want to make a change in your life, start now!
2. **Develop a Relentless Mindset.** In order to change your life, you need to develop mental toughness for when you

come across adversity and be relentless when you get knocked down.

3. **Create a Crystal Clear Vision.** Paint the picture of the life you want to see and live, then take action.

4. **Turn Adversity into Blessing in Disguise.** When times get rough, use the "Reframing Principle" and knock adversity on its ass.

5. **Develop Dynamic Habits.** Positive habits lead to more productivity. If you are not changing your habits, you are not open to changing yourself.

6. **Flexible Nutrition.** Understanding the basic principles of nutrition and your body's physiology can change your health and body composition.

7. **Realistic, Enjoyable, and Flexible Training.** If you cannot adhere to, or enjoy, your training program, you will not give it your all and will not maximize all the benefits of a well-rounded training program, along with a solid nutrition program.

8. **Four Pillars of Life.** Health, Wealth, Love, and Happiness are the key pillars to living the good life, along with a well-balanced lifestyle.

This book is the passageway of the eight strategies of BECOMING DYNAMIC that we have discovered along our journey, with help from our network, family, friends, mentors, coaches, and colleagues. By using these 8 proven strategies, you will not only become dynamic and experience The New Era of Fitness, you will also evolve and want to become a better all-around person each and every day.

We all have special and unique talents that we were blessed with. It's time to stop living in fear, following the status quo, and being average. We all have a calling and purpose in life; it's time you discover what that is. The time is now, and nothing is going to be given to you and nobody is going to feel sorry for you, so get out there take action, out work your competition, and change the world while being the best version of you! We will be right along your side doing the same, we promise! Let's Go!

CHAPTER 1

Now is the Time to Become Dynamic

"Out with the old and in with the new."

It's been a full decade since we started our fitness journey, and we have learned a lot. We've learned through self-experimentation, mentors, coaches, personal trainers, personal training clients, coaching clients online, having a life coach, our self-education, and higher learning institutes.

You see, we used to look at fitness under a microscope and think that life revolved around exercise and nutrition to the point where that's all we did and cared about. It would affect work, school, relationships, family functions, vacations, social events, you name it. That's what you call obsession, and fitness shouldn't put a strain on other important aspects in life.

It took us a decade to realize that solely focusing on exercise and nutrition won't lead to a long-term sustainable fitness journey. There's more to it. What we've learned these past ten years is you need to add lifestyle and mindset components to your fitness journey.

The Law of 33% in Your Fitness Program

As we go a bit deeper into exercise, nutrition, lifestyle, and mindset, there's a pretty cool law that has to do with mentorship:[1]

- 33% of the people you surround yourself with should be people less successful than you, so that you can help them, mentor them, and still learn a thing or two from them.
- 33% of the people you surround yourself with should be people on your level and the same playing field. So you can relate with them, share ideas, and continue to grow together.
- 33% of the people you surround yourself with should be people at elite levels, 10-20 years ahead of you so you can learn from them, avoid the same mistakes they made, and develop some of their habits.

This law off 33% adds up to 99% of your time and what your surroundings should be in order for you to achieve that elite level of success you are looking for in whatever endeavor you choose.

What if you applied this law of 33% into your fitness program?

Keep an open mind here. Think about 33% of your results coming through exercise, 33% of your results coming through nutrition, and 33% of your results coming through lifestyle and mindset. That makes up 99% of your results in fitness.

Gamifying your Fitness Journey

Think about when you were a kid; the majority of us liked playing video games, or others sorts of games, where you beat a level, were then rewarded, and then advanced to a higher level.

---

[1]   Tai Lopez. The Law of 33%. 2015. <https://www.youtube.com/watch?v=7bB_fVDlvhc>

Another mentor of ours, Chris Record, talks about gamifying your life[2]. He said "Turn your short term and long term goals into "Levels" and then focus every day on "Leveling Up!""

So, think about if you did this with your fitness journey? Imagine treating fitness like a game and having fun with it.

An example of gamifying your fitness journey would look like:

Level 1: Start by being active at least 30 minutes per day. Doesn't matter what it is; just be active for 30 min each day. If you accomplish this, then reward yourself and move onto the next level.

Level 2: Join a gym and make it there at least 3 days per week. No matter what, just make it there. If you accomplish this, then reward yourself and move onto the next level.

Level 3: Start by adding a structured exercise regime that consists of 4 days per week and follow it for a month or longer. If you accomplish this, then reward yourself and move onto the next level.

In this new era of fitness, it is time to start enjoying the process over the end product. Later in this book, you'll learn more about the habit loop, where we are rewarded for a small victory, constantly progressing over time, and advancing to the next level.

Fitness can't just be looked under a microscope anymore by just focusing on exercise and nutrition. The lifestyle and mindset components need to be applied in order for you to get results, constantly progress, enjoy the process, and create a long-term sustainable fitness journey around your life.

Times have changed, everything will continue to evolve, and the New Era of Fitness is here. It's up to you to adapt to it and evolve all around to better your health, wealth, love, and happiness.

Now we want you to go out and become Dynamic!

---

[2]   "Chris Record - GAMIFY LIFE Speech from Chris Record ... - Facebook." 2016. <https://www.facebook.com/ChrisRecord/videos/10155162109728289/>

Dynamic Tips

- Do not look at fitness under a microscope; look at the bigger picture and use the Law of 33%
- Gamify your fitness journey and have fun with it!
- Now is the time to take action and become dynamic; let's do it together!

Ready to start living dynamically? We have some game changing exercises in our Dynamic Lifestyle workbook for you. To get the workbook and enter The New Era of Fitness, go to **www.TheNewEraOfFitness.com/bonus**

CHAPTER 2

Develop a Relentless Mindset

"The two most important days in your life are the day you are born and the day you find out why."

– Mark Twain

Being Relentless is a state of mind that can give you strength to achieve, to survive, to overcome, and to be strong when others are not. It means craving the end result so intensely that the work becomes irrelevant in everything you do in life. In the movie *Lone Survivor*, Mark Wahlberg says, "You are always in the fight, never quit." That is the type of relentless mindset you need in order to survive in this world and get ahead. Nothing will ever be given to you, nor will anyone ever feel sorry for you; remember this statement, and you will be one step ahead of everyone else.

Don't Live in Fear

Something we have observed over the last 5 years is that society lives in fear. At the end of the day, fear is what holds us all back from what we really want to do, right? Think about how many people follow the path of least resistance, are comfortable with their current state, and fear failing. This is something we have paid very close attention to through ourselves, family members, friends, significant others, and clients we have coached. Not to mention, many people grew up seeing their parents live in fear while the school system tells them to play it safe. Growing up, we are taught to play it safe and follow the rules. That advice can actually be harmful when you start letting fear rule your life. Social rules and fears prevent you from achieving your dreams. Arnold Schwarzenegger once said, "Rules are meant to be broken, just don't break the law." It's normal to feel fear, fear should get your blood pumping full of excitement because you do not know what the outcome is going to be.

In the book *Relentless*, Tim Grover states:

Most people are the lion in the cage. Safe, tame, predictable, waiting for something to happen. But for humans, the cage isn't made of glass and steel bars; it's made of bad advice and low self-esteem and bullshit rules and tortured thinking about what you can't do or what you're supposed to do. It's molded around you by a lifetime of overthinking and overanalyzing and worrying about what could go wrong. Stay in the cage long enough, you forget those basic instincts.

Grover continues to point out how we put limits on ourselves because of fear. "When you feel fear, you recoil and put up a wall to protect yourself. Is there really a wall there? No, but you act as if there were. Now you can't go forward because of the wall. Put your hand through it, there's nothing there, you can walk straight through it. But if you stay behind that imaginary wall, you fail." This is 100% accurate, and we will be the first ones to tell you we have put up our fair share of walls along our journey. If you have a wall up currently, kick that wall down and take what's yours!

A simple formula presented in *Relentless* that we go by to avoid living in fear is: *Decide, Commit, Act, Experiment, Succeed, Be Relentless, and Repeat.* Make sure to write this down and put it somewhere visible so you can remind yourself how great you are and can be.

Comparing Yourself to Others

We don't care how good you think you are, or how great others think you are, you can always improve and should continue to improve 1% each and every day. Each day, you want to be a better version of yourself than yesterday in all areas of life. Being relentless means demanding more of yourself than anyone else could ever demand of you, knowing that every time you stop, you can still do more. Doing more is what separates winners from losers. Never ever compare yourself to others! We will repeat this again: never ever compare yourself to others! Be the best version of you, carve your own path, and write your own story, not somebody else's.

With social media being so powerful these days, we cannot tell you how many times we have had clients compare themselves to other people's body images on Instagram. Social media can be very misleading for the fitness industry and can really do a number psychologically. When we started our business, we compared ourselves with other elite coaches and bodybuilders; we had no right to and we are so glad we snapped out of that kind of mindset. It is toxic, plain and simple. You have to stop, think, and ask yourself, why the hell am I comparing myself to other people when my only competition is the person I see in the mirror each day?

Everyone is born with talents. We truly believe though that talent without hard work means nothing, and talent can be outworked by someone who is driven and persistent. You have to use the talent you are given; so many people let their talents go to waste...We love this quote by Michael Jordan, "Everyone has talent, but ability takes hard work."

Developing Mental Toughness

"The first secret to mental toughness, as simple as it may sound, is to recognize and embrace the power of choice and how that power can shape our lives."

– Mark Devine

We all have thousands of choices to make in our lives each and every day. The choices we make are what ultimately dictate our health, wealth, love, and happiness. These are the Four Pillars of Life, and we will get more in depth with these later in the book. When we lost our father in 2004, lost our grandmother, and lost part of our mom, we had the choice to either give up on life or keep pushing forward. We had our moments where we got into trouble with the law and we could have kept going down that path, but we didn't. We remembered where we came from and how our parents raised us. We knew we had too much potential to offer the world rather than throw it all away.

We didn't have a secret formula for mental toughness when we were going through all these tragedies; we developed mental toughness along the way by making mistakes and learning from them. At some point, you have to adapt to every situation you are in. What we can tell you is that we mastered 3 things that really helped us mentally and emotionally get through challenging times. Those 3 things are as follows:

1. Make the Right Choice
    Don't put all your eggs in one basket. Take your time to identify all the pros and cons to each choice you have and trust your instincts and refer to your core values.

2. Manage Your Stress
    Stress is stress, and it is not going anywhere anytime soon. Learn to manage your stress on a daily basis and do not ever let it overtake you and your emotions. Try breathing techniques, walks, yoga, podcasts, words of affirmations, and sometimes just chill out.

3. Create Emotional Resiliency
    We are all emotional human beings and our emotions can get the best of us. It's ok to cry and let those sorrows out, just don't let them override what you are focused on. Learn to master your emotions.

Cultivating a relentless mindset is not an overnight task. Vision, focus, discipline, belief in self, humility, and the pursuit of greatness are all the products of developed emotional intelligence, a fine art that requires a lot of practice. Nothing great happens overnight; be patient and develop that relentless mindset that is inside of you. You were put on this earth to be great and make an impact!

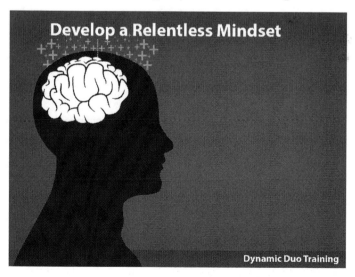

Dynamic Tips

- You are always in the fight, never quit, be relentless and keeping fighting.
- Do not live in fear! Learn to step outside of your comfort zone and break some rules, but not laws.
- Comparing yourself to others is toxic. Carve your own path and live a life worth telling a story about.
- Develop mental toughness using our three tips.

Do you want to learn how to create a Relentless Mindset?
We have some game changing exercises in our Dynamic Lifestyle workbook for you. To get the workbook and enter The New Era of Fitness, go to
www.TheNewEraOfFitness.com/bonus

CHAPTER 3

Create a Crystal Clear Vision

"People are capable, at any time in their lives, of doing what they dream of."
– Paulo Coelho, The Alchemist

A vision is about creating a short statement or painting a picture that will guide you over the next 3 to 5 years, or even longer. It should be specific enough to say something about what you will do and equally what you will not do. We truly believe a strong vision represents your Identity, Calling, and Assignment in life.[3] Your vision should be capable of driving you to achieve a common goal and be motivational so that you have a constant reminder of what you are trying to achieve when the going gets tough.

Without a vision, a goal is like a ship without a rudder and is in danger of drifting aimlessly and can eventually sink. Joel A. Baker said, "Vision without action is merely a dream. Action without vision just passes the time. Vision with action can change the world." Many people lack a clear vision, and so they tend to jump from task to task without a clear understanding of what bonds the individual actions together and/or the value created by the individual actions. Your vision should provide the cornerstone for everything that you do and your goals in life.

---

[3]   "H3 Leadership — Brad Lomenick." 2015. <http://www.bradlomenick.com/h3-leadership/>

Through the years, we have learned that if you think about strategy (the "how") too early, it will actually inhibit your vision (the "what") and block you from thinking as big as you need to think. What you need is a vision that is so BIG, it scares you, that is compelling, not only to others, but to you as well. If it's not compelling, you won't have the motivation to stay the course and you won't be able to recruit others to help you.

When we first started our business Dynamic Duo Training, we had no vision whatsoever. We thought we did, but in all honesty, we had no clue. Looking back, we often wonder if things would be different within our business today if we'd have a vision from the start. Unfortunately you cannot go back in time, and that was just one of our big mistakes as young entrepreneurs. We can tell you one thing though, we both absolutely always thought big or go home with our business. If you are a young entrepreneur, we highly suggest spending some time and figuring out what your vision and overall big picture is. Figure out your Identity, Calling, and Assignment in life first and that will shed some light. Having a clear vision is so vital for businesses, health and fitness, and goals in general.

When it comes to health and fitness and creating a vision, think bigger picture and longevity here. Many people want to get results quickly rather than take their time to do it right. We try telling our clients to look at it as a marathon, not a sprint. Set short, medium, and long term goals that are realistic, then take action on these goals, and this will make your vision come to life.

Identity, Calling, and Assignment

These are components we struggled with at an early age, especially when we lost our father and went through some dark times. Once we came across the amazing book by Brad Lomenick titled *H3 Leadership: Be Humble, Stay Hungry, Always Hustle* and listened to a podcast episode with Lewis Howes and Brad Lomenick, a light bulb struck us. We finally knew what our Identity, Calling, and Assignments were in life, and this made our vision crystal clear about what we wanted to do with our business and ourselves going forward. If you take a look at the picture below, you will get a better understanding of how you can break down what your Identity, Calling, and Assignments are.

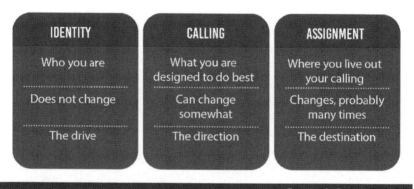

Identity: You have to understand that your Identity does not change. For an example of our Identity: We are Eric and Chris Martinez, born in Santa Rosa, California, sons of Miguel and Marie Martinez. Now you try it, and understand this will not change.

Calling: Your calling is what you were designed to do best in this world, how are you going to serve others and make an impact. This can change, but ultimately, this is what will really help you gain clarity and direction on your vision. For an example of our Calling: We are designed to serve and help others change their health, fitness, and lifestyle habits. We are here to motivate, educate, and inspire people to change their lives.

Assignment: For us, the assignment is what really makes this all exciting. Your assignment can change, and most likely will, but it's ultimately where you live out your calling. For an example of our Assignment: We are currently living out our calling in Orange County, California. Right now, our assignment is to help change as many lives as we possibly can while scaling our business and reaching a bigger audience. We know our assignment will change and we will embrace that, but the exciting part is we do not have a final destination.

Once you have identified all of these components about yourself, write down your vision and see if it becomes even clearer than before. You become what you envision yourself being.

"A vision is not just a dream. A powerful vision emerges when we couple our dreams with a set of clear goals. Without both, we are apt to wander in a clueless and purposeless fog, because a dream without goals is just a fantasy. And fantasies are the bad kind of visions, the hallucinogenic kind, not the real kind."

– Lewis Howes

If you really want to be great at anything, you have got to have a crystal clear vision of exactly what you want, why you want it, and when you want it to happen. All of our amazing mentors that we look up to have all done this and created a crystal clear vision. When we first started our online training and nutrition business, we looked up so much to our mentor and coach Layne Norton to the point we wanted to be just like him. After some years of trial and error within our business, learning from other mentors and discovering our Identity, Calling, and Assignment, we knew we couldn't be Layne Norton and we didn't have any right to. We had to be our own versions of Eric and Chris Martinez, run our business our way, continue to get 1% better each and every day, and we couldn't be any happier with that outcome thus far.

Think about how many athletes grow up idolizing legendary professionals; we know we did. How many of us wanted to be the next Michael Jordan, Serena Williams, Ronda Rousey, Peyton Manning, and Barry Bonds? We are sure many people in the world envisioned themselves being like these hall of famer athletes, but realize they cannot at some point in their lives. You can absolutely be great like them with hard work and talent, but chances are you will never be who they are, what they accomplished, and have their mindset and visions. You have to create your own vision because you have a different Identity, Calling and Assignment. We are all meant to write a different story.

Staying Focused

Our mentor Tai Lopez once advised, "If you cannot stay focused with your vision and work ethic, you will fail." For some reason, that really stuck with us and made us realize the importance of staying focused in this crazy world we live in today. Not only within our business, but as people as well, it is important to stay focused. Think of all the distractions out there with social media, the status quo of working a 9-5 job, politics, religion, the list goes on. It's very easy to get distracted in today's society. Not to mention, attention spans are at an all-time low. We are guilty of not staying focused from time to time; we are human after all.

In *Focus: The Hidden Driver of Excellence*, Daniel Goleman suggests a different perspective about a wandering mind. "Every variety of attention has its uses. The very fact that about half of our thoughts are daydreams suggests there may well be some advantage to a mind that can entertain the fanciful. We might revise our own thinking about a "wandering mind," by considering that rather than wandering *away* from what counts, we may well be wandering *toward* something of value." Just stop and think for a minute how many times you have been working on something important and your mind either wanders off daydreaming or your attention is drawn towards an attractive person walking by? Come on, we are all guilty of this; it is normal human nature. We are both guilty as charged on this one, but we find that this happens too often with everyone in general. Just think how much more productive you'd be on a project if you were to focus a bit more and get rid of all the distractions around you.

Some simple steps to stay focused when working on something important can be as follows:

- Turn your phone or notifications off, this way not even a ring tone sets your brain off
- Turn off all social media windows and email on your laptops
- Play some relaxing music to get your body and mind relaxed
- Choose an appropriate work setting. If you know you lose focus at a coffee shop, don't go to a coffee shop. Go to a public library.

At the end of the day, we are all responsible for our own actions and how we manage our time. You can make the excuse that you cannot focus. Staying focused is on the top of our list in regards to getting shit done and bringing our crystal clear vision to life. Your vision will suffer if you cannot gain control of your overall focus. Remember, a vision without any action and clarity is just a dream. Take the time to develop a crystal clear vision of what you want in life.

Dynamic Tips

- Write down 2-3 visions and share them with people who will give you honest feedback.
- Take your time to figure out your Identity, Calling, and Assignment. Then place these somewhere visual in your home so they are a constant reminder.
- Envision the life you want to live and think big.
- Stay FOCUSED and continue to experiment with what works best for you.

Do you want to learn how to create a Crystal Clear Vision?
We have some game changing exercises in our Dynamic
Lifestyle workbook for you. To get the workbook and enter
The New Era of Fitness, go to
www.TheNewEraOfFitness.com/bonus

CHAPTER 4

Turn Adversity into Blessings in Disguise

"We all get knocked down. How quickly we get up is what separates us."
– Darren Hardy

We often wonder how life would really be without any type of adversity or obstacles to overcome. If you really stop and think about it, adversity and overcoming obstacles are what make life exciting. Life without any adversity would be a linear road that everyone follows; there would be no challenges, thus no reward. Who would want to live in a world like that? We know we sure wouldn't.

As you learned in the preface, adversity has always been in our life and vocabulary; we are no strangers to it. Losing our father, grandmother, and a piece of our mother was the most difficult challenge ever. Overcoming adversity has made us mentally, emotionally, and spiritually stronger individuals. Whenever you lose a parent or family member, life is never the same. You have to understand that, move forward, and adapt to the best of your ability. There are tragedies every single day around the world and never any answers as to why they happen. Adversity is rough and can suck you dry, but if you can overcome it, we promise you it will make you a stronger person overall.

Our 30 Day Notice

We will never forget the obstacle we had to overcome during the month of June, 2016. We still remember getting the email towards the end of the month in May while we were on vacation in Miami. It hit us like a ton of bricks, and we tried so hard not to put our focus and energy towards it until our vacation was over.

We were living in a 3 bedroom townhome in Orange County, California, and had our own office for our business and our own private gym built into our garage where we trained a handful of clients, produced content for videos, and trained ourselves. Everything was going amazing there where we lived, but one stormy day in Miami while on vacation, we received an email from our landlord indicating he wanted to sell his townhome. There was nothing we could do to control this situation, and we didn't want this to ruin our current vacation.

When we returned back home from Miami, we literally had 30 days to move everything out and find a new place to rent. We were so overwhelmed and bummed, we just couldn't grasp why this was happening to us. We said to ourselves, "Haven't we been put through enough already? Why do we always get hit with these horrible obstacles?" We sat there for a day or two, depressed and angry, but after talking to our family, friends, and mentors, we just accepted the reality of it - it was another curveball thrown our way. We said to ourselves, "This is happening for a reason. It is a test from God, and there is something bigger and better out there for us. Only we can dig ourselves out of this hole, nobody is going to feel sorry for us, so we need to stop feeling sorry for ourselves." We realized there were two things we could do in this situation:

1. Curl up into a ball in a dark room and cry about feeling sorry for ourselves, being angry at the world, and letting this curveball defeat us.

2. We step up to the plate and smash that curveball out of the park and prevail!

Our next step was going back to the drawing board to look at our overall vision, come up with a game plan to execute in the next 30 days, and use the Reframing Principle. Below we will teach you some of the Reframing Principles we learned from Internet Marketing Guru, Chris Record. We tried to find another 3 bedroom home to accommodate all of our needs, prices ranges, and more, but it became extremely difficult to find a decent place, and time was ticking. After 21 days of searching for another house, we came to the conclusion that the cards were not on our side with this one. If it was meant to be, we would have found something that we were looking for. We are firm believers that God has a plan for all of us, and we realized we were not meant to find another 3 bedroom home.

Our next step was to find a 2 bedroom apartment, sell our entire gym equipment that was well over 8k, and just move on with life. We luckily found a very nice 2 bedroom apartment in Anaheim, California. We ended up selling our entire gym and a ton of our furniture all within a week. We still remember when the first piece of our gym equipment was sold. It was so hard letting it go and accepting what the reality was, we worked so damn hard for that gym and we knew we were not going to get back what we paid for all of it.

After selling our entire gym, the rest was history and we moved to our new place. We look at the adversity and obstacle we came over as a blessing in disguise. The blessing is that there is something bigger and better out there for us, and that is exactly where our mindset is currently. To use the adversity we faced and overcame as a blessing to push forward with life has made us even stronger individuals overall. None of this would have been possible if we did not believe in ourselves or have faith.

The Reframing Principle

We are always going to be the kind of guys who give credit where credit is due. We first found out about the reframing principle from an entrepreneur, Chris Record. We were at a business seminar, and Chris Record was a guest speaker talking about his life story and all of the adversity he faced and overcame, such as losing his marriage, filing for bankruptcy, and treating his child that had several medical conditions. Our jaws literally dropped when we heard his entire story and learned about how much adversity he overcame. It really goes to show that when you think you have it bad, you really have no idea what others have been through or are currently going through.

Chris talked about using the Reframing Principle. When you are faced with adversity, how fast can you bounce back? Below you will see the main bullet points on what the Reframing Principle consists of:

- Learn how to reframe adversity into blessings and opportunities in disguise
- Instead of saying "I can't", say "How can I?"
- You have to believe the impossible is possible
- Believe in yourself!

If we would have known about this Reframing Principle when we were younger, we could have really saved ourselves some heartache and mistakes along the way. Whenever you are facing adversity, try and use the Reframing Principle to give yourself a different outlook on why this is happening to you and how you can overcome it.

You Have to Believe and Have Faith

At the end of the day, you have to believe you can overcome any type of adversity, no matter what is thrown your way. If you cannot believe nor have any faith, adversity will most likely get the best of

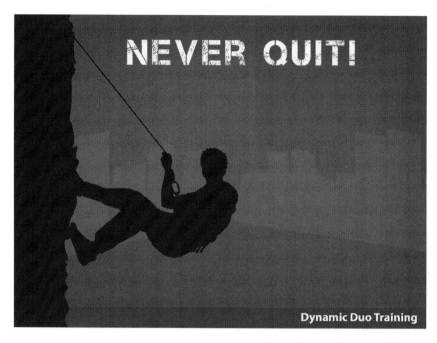

NEVER QUIT!

Dynamic Duo Training

you. You have to be relentless and knock that adversity on its ass! As we said earlier in this chapter, adversity is what makes life exciting and keeps the adrenaline going. Yes, tragedies happen from time to time to good people, but that is out of your control. You can only control what you can; there is no reason to stress what you cannot. Next time you are faced with adversity, welcome it, learn from it, knock it on its ass, and enjoy the ride!

Dynamic Tips

- Everyone has had and will face adversity, it's part of life, prepare yourself as best as you can
- Use the Reframing Principle when faced with adversity
- Believe in yourself and have Faith

- Never ever quit
- Welcome it, learn from it, knock it on its ass, and enjoy the ride

Ready to turn your adversities into blessings?
We have some game changing exercises in our Dynamic
Lifestyle workbook for you. To get the workbook and enter
The New Era of Fitness, go to
www.TheNewEraOfFitness.com/bonus

CHAPTER 5

Develop Dynamic Habits

"Motivation is what gets you started. Habit is what keep you going."
– Jim Rohn

We have a confession to make…when we first started our fitness journey, all we wanted was the end result and that was to have chiseled abs, a superhero-comic book looking muscular chest, a back bigger than the state of Texas, and of course, the massive guns (arms) for the ladies.

We never thought about building good behavioral habits, laying down the bricks for a strong foundation, creating systems, gaining knowledge for longevity within fitness, and most importantly, enjoying the actual process, not just focusing on the end product.

You see, getting your dream physique is just an end result from a good exercise and nutrition program.

But without building good behavioral habits and laying down the bricks for a strong foundation…there is no system created for a long term and sustainable fitness journey.

Habits are even important in sports, as Super Bowl winning coach Tony Dungy can attest to. He wanted to simplify the game to reduce the margin for error. Instead of drilling a bunch of formations into his player's heads, he selected only a handful. He then made his team practice them relentlessly until the behaviors became second nature.

From this, he was able to create faster, sleeker teams that ran on the fuel of habits, not just relying on talent.

Think about Michael Jordan, Phil Jackson, and the Chicago Bulls. Phil created the triangle offense, which in turn became a habit for the team to run. Every opponent knew they were going to run the triangle, but did they stop Michael and the Bulls? Hardly ever.

Researchers at Duke University found that more than 40 percent of actions people performed each day weren't actual decisions, but habits.[4] Habits are everything and in our opinion, they are the key to success.

Let's dive into how to build good behavioral habits.

The Habit Loop

To form a habit, there are 3 steps:[5]

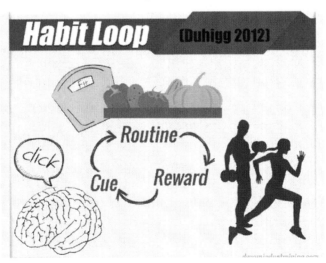

---

4   Neal, David T., Wendy Wood, and Jeffrey M. Quinn. "Habits—A repeat performance." Current Directions in Psychological Science 15.4 (2006): 198–202.

5   "The Power of Habit by Charles Duhigg." 2012. <http://charlesduhigg.com/the-power-of-habit/>

Step 1: There is a CUE, a trigger, that tells your brain to go into automatic mode and which habit to use

Step 2: Then there is a ROUTINE, which can be physical, mental, or emotional

Step 3: Finally, there is a REWARD, which helps your brain figure out if this particular loop is worth remembering for the future

Over time, this habit loop - Cue, routine, and reward becomes more automatic. The cue and the reward become intertwined until a powerful sense of anticipation and craving emerges.

Now, if we take exercise and nutrition as an example, the reason it's so hard to build good habits is because once you develop a routine of sitting on the couch rather than exercising or grabbing donuts at your leisure instead of having a healthy-balanced meal, those patterns always remain in your head.

However, if you were to program your brain and teach it new neurological routines that overpower those poor behavioral habits (donuts and sitting on the couch) and apply the habit loop…you can force those bad tendencies to the back burner and create new ones.

Exercise Example:

Step 1: The Cue - You're tired of seeing your body image in the mirror everyday when you shower, but you're too tired to work out after a long day of work

Step 2: The Routine - You start bringing your exercise clothes to work with you and go straight to the gym instead of coming home and getting relaxed

Step 3: The Reward - You consistently start attending the gym and exercising for 2-3 months, your body starts changing, and you start to like what you see in the mirror

Nutrition example:

Step 1: The Cue - You're tired of feeling and looking like crap from all the eating out, snacking, and junk foods you're consuming, but you have no desire to grocery shop or cook

Step 2: The Routine - You start by hiring a chef that comes to your house once per week, does all your grocery shopping, and cooks you healthy and delicious meals, or perhaps you go the meal prep service route and have healthy-delicious foods delivered to your home

Step 3: The Reward - You start to have more energy day to day, you feel better at work, you work harder, and you are even inspired to start exercising

Always remember...Starting off with good habits is everything and builds a solid foundation to have success within your fitness journey.

Cue and Reward Yourself From Now On

In 2002, researchers at New Mexico State University wanted to understand why people habitually exercise.[6] 266 subjects were studies who performed at least 3 days per week of exercise. What they found was that many of them had started running or lifting weights almost on a whim, or because they suddenly had free time or wanted to deal with unexpected stresses in their lives.

However, the reason they continued and why it became a habit was because of a specific reward they started to crave.

---

[6]   Finlay, Krystina A., David Trafimow, and Aimee Villarreal. "Predicting Exercise and Health Behavioral Intentions: Attitudes, Subjective Norms, and Other Behavioral Determinants1." *Journal of Applied Social Psychology* 32.2 (2002): 342-356.

In one group, 92 percent of people said they habitually exercised because it made them feel good. In the other group, 67 percent of people said that exercising gave them a sense of accomplishment.

If you put this into a real life example, say you want to work out every morning for 30 minutes, it's essential that you choose a simple cue like leaving your gym clothes out, so right when you wake up, the clothes laid out triggers your brain to get ready and workout. Once you have your simple cue, set a reward for yourself, such as eating something non-traditional like a piece of chocolate or a small treat just to get your sense of accomplishment.

Some other forms of rewards you can do are:

A. Try picking a habit you want to start, like removing processed foods, then rate yourself on a scale from 1-5 (1 being " a poor job" and 5 being "an amazing job") at the end of the week. If you got a 4 or 5 then reward yourself, if you got a 1 or 2 then try the habit over again next week, and if you got a 3, then that's a decision you have to make yourself as to whether you should be rewarded or not. What this could look like is removing 2-3 processed food items a week. If we are successful with it for a week straight, we rate ourselves a 5 and then have a small indulgence meal as a reward.

B. There are apps now where you can give yourself points or stars after each task that you performed. Simply use a new habit as a task, experiment with it for a week, and then rate yourself daily or weekly with the app. Depending on the total points or stars you get in a week or month, reward yourself with something. Some really good apps are:

1. **Balanced-Goals & Habits motivation:** Struggling to make time for all the little things that matter? Join over 500,000 others who use this app to stay motivated and focused on what's really important in life. (http://balancedapp.com/)

2. **Habit List-Create good habits, break bad ones:**
   Create good habits and break unhealthy ones to build a
   better you. (http://habitlist.com/)
3. **Habits Pro-Organizer for goals, task and health:**
   Looking for a new year and new you? This app helps
   with workouts, time management, mindset, and more.
   (http://tracknshareapp.com/habits-pro/)

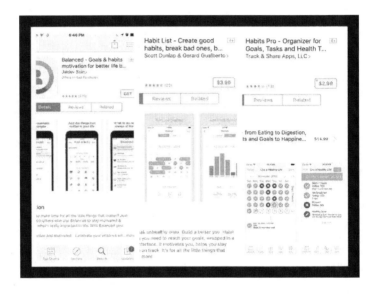

C. In the context of exercise and nutrition, give yourself a
   monthly total of 20 points. You assess yourself, or someone
   else assesses you, on a 10 point scale in these 2 categories.
   You don't have to maintain a certain ranking in one category,
   you just have to maintain a certain total. So let's say it's a 15
   point total out of 20 that you need to attain for the month.
   Maybe you have a really good month at the gym and get
   all your workouts in, and that gives you 10 full points for
   your exercise category; however, your nutrition was off due

to traveling or very busy work week, so you give yourself a 5 for that category, well that turns out to be a total of 15 points! Now you need to reward yourself. This is a very simple and non-technical way of creating good habits.

Just remember the habit loop and most importantly see what sparks the cue for you, and then make sure to reward yourself some way.

Sets and Reps

"A habit is a practice shaped by behavior or daily action that helps turn ideals into action, principles into practice, and concepts into concrete. Habits allow for someone to actually implement ideas that last into his or her life. Habits create standard operating procedures in your life and a re the fuel to get to the finish line."

– Brad Lomenick, H3 Leadership:
Stay Hungry. Be Humble. Always Hustle.

Want to change your body composition? Create sound fitness habits in your life. Want to incorporate more nutritious foods into your diet? Create good nutritional habits. Want to get better at squatting or deadlifting? Create good training habits through sets and reps.

If you want to get good at anything in life, it just takes sets and reps. Arnold Schwarzenegger shared this realization in his book Total Recall. This is how he became Mr. Olympia 7 times, how he became good at real estate, how he became a blockbuster actor, and how he became a governor.

Sets and reps are just practice, which turns into habits, which turns into success.

Like we said earlier, habits are everything. Creating good habits will take you far in any endeavor in life, and we are prime examples of habits taking you far in your fitness journey.

Dynamic Tips

- Write down 2-3 Habits you want to change right now, and put them somewhere visual to constantly remind you each day.
- Refer to the "Habit Loop" as your first step to improve a Habit.
- Cue and Reward yourself on these Habits when you improve them.
- Use an App if needed; there are plenty of great suggestions above.

Ready to develop Dynamic Habits? We have some game changing exercises in our Dynamic Lifestyle workbook for you. To get the workbook and enter The New Era of Fitness, go to
www.TheNewEraOfFitness.com/bonus

CHAPTER 6

Flexible Nutrition

"Let food be thy medicine, and medicine be thy food."

– Hippocrates

The fitness industry is full of diets, full of extremists, full of people who claim their diet works because of X,Y, Z; full of bad information…you get the picture, right?

The problem with the issues above is there's hardly any kind of data out of the scientific literature to backup their claims. In this new era of fitness, we are students of science who use data from top studies within the health community. To be 100% honest, we're not trying to sell you on anything. After reading this chapter, if you still want to try other diets, then go right ahead and do so; to each their own. All we're trying to present is a nutrition system that has worked for us, our clients, many other people, and has science to back it up.

Before we get into what flexible nutrition is, we need to lay down the bricks of learning how to properly advance to higher nutrition levels.

It's like the legendary UCLA basketball coach, John Wooden said, "Be quick, but don't hurry."

There's no need to hurry or rush advancing your nutrition levels. You can absolutely be quick in the learning curve if you catch on quickly and build good habits, but never hurry.

Consistency, Adherence, and Habits

Like Gary Vaynerchuck says, "Be authentic 24/7/365." We want to be authentic and real with you about how badly we messed up in the beginning of our nutrition programs. When we started our very first nutrition program, all we wanted was the end result, and that was to have an amazing physique. We made so many mistakes and wasted a lot of money. When it came to fads and trends you name it, we did it.

We never thought about building good behavioral habits, laying down the bricks for a strong foundation, creating systems, gaining knowledge for longevity within nutrition, and most importantly, enjoying the actual process, not just the product.

Without building good behavioral habits and laying down the bricks for a strong foundation… there is no system created for a long term and sustainable nutrition program and thus, no results are attained.

Once you have these good behavioral habits built, this will make being consistent and adherent within your nutrition program that much easier.

So that's why we put consistency, adherence, and habits at the forefront because if you don't get these principles down, then the rest of the tools you gain won't help.

Beginner's Stage

Before we delve into this, just keep in mind that consistency and adherence will always be at the forefront for any nutrition program. If you can't see yourself doing this nutrition program for days, weeks, months and years, then you need to re-evaluate the components of the program to see what's working and what's not and fine tune it until you increase your adherence and consistency.

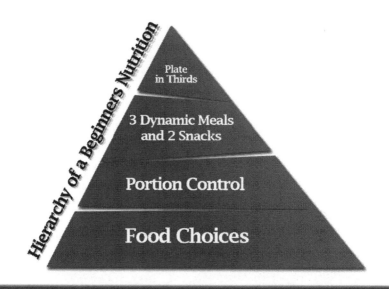

With our experience working with over a 1,000 clients, being mentored by other experts, going through higher education institutes, and our own self education, we feel if you are brand new to all of this fitness stuff, you should follow the nutrition recommendations below to build a solid foundation:

Plate of Thirds Rule

We want you to close your eyes and picture you have a squeaky clean-white dinner plate in front of you.

Now, we want you to divide that plate into thirds. Each of your meals should be comprised of a high quality protein source, complex carbohydrate source, and a healthy fat source.[7]

---

[7]   Whitney E, Rolfes S. Understanding Nutrition. 13th edition. 2013

Now that you have your plate in thirds, we want you to have a high quality protein source covering a third of the plate. Protein sources can be:

- Chicken
- Fish
- Eggs
- Beef
- Whey, egg, pea, rice protein powders
- Dairy

The next third of the plate should consist of a complex carbohydrate source. Complex carbohydrate sources can consist of:

- Brown or white rice
- Oats
- Whole wheat or Whole grain breads
- Potatoes (however botanically classified as vegetables)
- Beans

Lastly, you want a healthy fat source covering that final third of the plate. Healthy fat sources can consist of:

- Nuts/Seeds
- Almond/Peanut butter
- Olive oil/Coconut oil
- Animal fats (egg yolks, red meat, fatty fish)
- Avocados

Each of your meals should comprise of a high quality protein source, complex carbohydrate source, and a healthy fat source.

Your plate could look like:

- A grilled chicken breast
- Sticky white rice
- Steamed vegetables with a side of roasted almonds

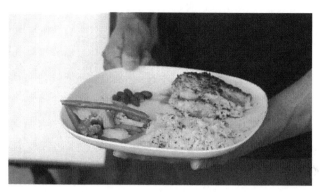

3 Dynamic Meals and 2 Snacks

Next up on the hierarchy of nutrition, we have 3 Dynamic Meals and 2 snacks. When we say "Dynamic Meals," we are referring to larger-core meals. A good way to look at this is your typical breakfast, lunch, and dinner meals. When you have these larger-core meals, you generally want to spread them out about 4-6 hours apart. An example of this would look like:

Dynamic Meal 1: 8 a.m.
Dynamic Meal 2: 1 p.m.
Dynamic Meal 3: 6 p.m.

Moving on to incorporating 2 snacks, we like to advocate more of a higher protein type of snack. If you have your 3 Dynamic Meals, the average person will usually consume approximately 20-40g of protein at each meal. If you consume the latter part of that at each meal (approx. 40g) you're coming very close to the recommended dietary allowance (RDA) of protein intake which is 0.8g/lb.[8]

But what if we threw in some more protein? A study by Jose Antonio and colleagues showed more protein intake has the following benefits[9]:

- Increased satiety (feeling more full)
- Increased TEF (Thermic Effect of Food; your body works harder to break protein down and thus expends more calories)
- More muscle mass retention

This is where adding in 2 higher protein snacks can be beneficial, with options such as:

- Greek yogurt
- Whey, egg, pea, and rice protein powder shakes
- Beef jerky
- Turkey slices

So if you add 2 snacks in between your 3 Dynamic Meals, it would look like this:

Dynamic Meal 1: 8 a.m.
Snack 1: 11 a.m.

Dynamic Meal 2: 1 p.m.
Snack 2: 4 p.m.

---

[8]   Institute of medicine. Dietary reference intakes for energy, carbohydrates, fiber, fat, protein and amino acids. 2005

[9]   Antonio, Jose et al. "A high protein diet (3.4 g/kg/d) combined with a heavy resistance training program improves body composition in healthy trained men and women—a follow-up investigation." *Journal of the International Society of Sports Nutrition* 12.1 (2015): 1.

Dynamic Meal 3: 6 p.m.

In a 24 hour period, you should try and aim for 3 Dynamic meals and 2 higher protein source snacks.

Portion Control

Before we get to the third tier, do us a favor and pat yourself on the back because you're moving along down the pyramid within your nutrition.

Now that you have a sense of what your plate should look like (plate in thirds), how many meals you should have (3 dynamic meals and 2 snacks), we want to teach you how to portion out your serving sizes within this plate that's divided into thirds. This rule is called the "Precision Nutrition Control" rule.[10]

For women, the portion of protein at primary meals should be the size of the palm of your open hand. For men, we recommend two palm sized portions with each meal.

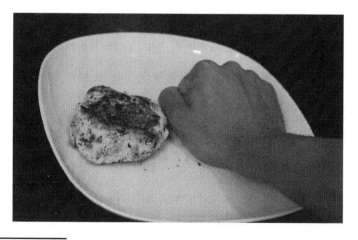

---

[10]   "Precision Nutrition: Nutrition Coaching and Certification." 2003.
   <http://www.precisionnutrition.com/>

For women, the portion of carbohydrates at primary meals should be 1 cupped hand sized. For men, we recommend 2 cupped hand sized portions.

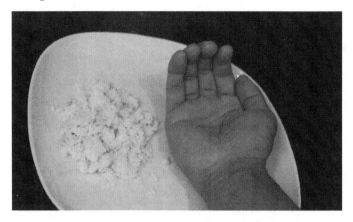

For women, we recommend 1 thumb sized portion of extra fats. For men, we recommend 2 thumb sized portions of extra fats. If the portion sizes are slightly bigger than your thumb, don't stress over it.

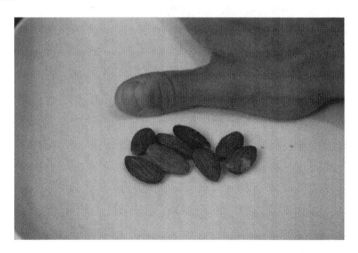

It's important to keep in mind that these are just general rules and recommendations. If you are looking to gain muscle mass, your portions may want to be a bit bigger and vice versa, if you are dieting, portion sizes may be smaller.

Another great way to keep yourself accountable for your portion sizes and making sure you're including protein, carbs, and fats into your meals is to take photos of your meals and analyze them.

Make a folder in your computer with the dates and label them Monday through Friday. Each day you will take pics of your meals, save them, review them at the end of the day, and then try improving upon them the following day.

As long as you're portioning your meals out with the above recommendations and taking pictures of your meals, you will be doing just fine within your nutrition program.

Food Choices

Alright…3 tiers down on the pyramid, and there's one left to go over that's just as important as the others - food selection.

People decide what to eat, when to eat, how much to eat, and whether to eat in highly personal ways based on a complex interaction of genetic, behavioral, or social factors rather than an awareness of nutrition's importance to health.[11]

As you might expect, the number one reason most people choose certain foods is taste; they like the flavor. Other reasons people select certain foods are:

- Out of habit, like eating cereal every morning for breakfast
- Cultural reasons

[11] Cohen, Robin A, and Patricia F Adams. "Use of the Internet for health information: United States, 2009." Jul. 2011.

- Social interactions
- Availability, convenience, and economy

Food choices are huge within a nutrition program because there are foods that are considered "higher energy density," which consist of:

- Higher calorie foods
- Processed and highly palatable foods (more sugar, carbs and fats)
- Overall less nutrient value for the body

On the other hand, your nutrition program should predominantly consist of whole and minimally refined foods, which consist of:

- Lower calorie foods
- Higher quality protein, fruits, vegetables, healthy fats, and complex carbohydrates
- Overall more nutrient value for the body

When you're putting together your plate in thirds and 3 dynamic meals and 2 snacks, the majority of your food choices should be of whole and minimally refined foods that are going to provide a lot of nutrient density to your body (see healthy food choice examples above under "plate in thirds" discussion).

Intermediate Stage:

Now whip out your phone, take a quick selfie, pat yourself on the back because you just graduated from your beginners based nutrition program, learned the fundamentals of nutrition, gained some great behavioral habits, and now you're ready to step up your game and be an intermediate.

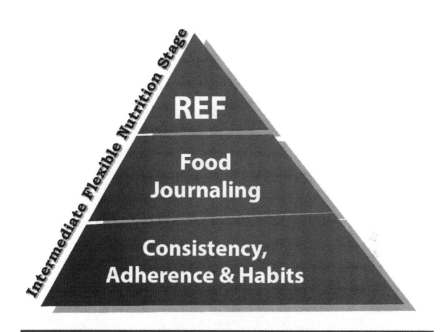

Like we touched on in the beginning of this section, we feel after working with so many clients, that the beginner's stage is really one of the more important stages in your nutrition program. If you can get past the beginners stage and gain all of the tools that we just discussed, then the intermediate and advanced stages are just icing on the cake, and who knows, you may just be happy with your results from all the tools you learned in the beginners stage. Whenever you want to take your physique to the next level, then you can apply the tools we will teach you from the intermediate and advanced stages.

If you mastered the beginner's tools, then you should follow the intermediate nutrition recommendations below:

Food Journaling

Weight loss occurs because of the low energy intake. Any diet can produce weight loss, at least temporarily, if intake is restricted.[12]

The real value of a diet is determined by its ability to maintain weight loss and support good health over the long term. The goal is not simply weight loss, but health gains. Most of these fad diets cannot support optimal health over time. In fact, these fad diets can create or exacerbate health problems such as eating disorders, etc.[13]

Some of these nutrition programs are just fads and will do more damage than good. They rarely support good health and habits over the long term.

A 2005 study from *The New England Journal of Medicine* showed that "lifestyle modification" practices that include keeping daily records of food and calorie intake and physical activity resulted in significant weight loss. These results also confirm previous reports from Klein, Sheard, Pi-Sunyer et al. 2004. Of the benefits of lifestyle modification (i.e., keeping daily records of food and calorie intake and physical activity) used alone for inducing weight loss.[14]

Moreover, a 1993 study from *The Journal of Behavioral Therapy* showed self-monitoring is necessary for successful weight control. Specifically, the monitoring of: Any food eaten, all foods eaten, time food was eaten, quantity of food eaten, and grams of fat consumed was positively correlated with weight change, while no monitoring at all was negatively associated with weight change.[15]

---

[12]   NHLBI 1998; Wing 2001; Jakicic 2001
[13]   Whitney E, Rolfes S. Understanding Nutrition. 13th edition. 2013
[14]   Wadden, Thomas A et al. "Randomized trial of lifestyle modification and pharmacotherapy for obesity." *New England Journal of Medicine* 353.20 (2005): 2111-2120.
[15]   Baker, Raymond C, and Daniel S Kirschenbaum. "Self-monitoring may be necessary for successful weight control." *Behavior Therapy* 24.3 (1993): 377-394.

The above studies support why flexible nutrition and tracking your food intake works. You have complete control over what you are putting into your body, you're not excluding food groups, you are not suffering, you are simply counting your macronutrients, eating whole and minimally refined foods, getting adequate micronutrient intakes, and transitioning it into a lifestyle.

REF...Realistic, Enjoyable, and Flexible

Our coach, mentor, and colleague, Eric Helms, talked about REF in his Muscle and Strength Video Series.[16] He talked about REF in relation to planning. Before you plan out your exercise program and weekly training schedule, you need to take these 3 factors into consideration:

R - Realistic
E - Enjoyable
F - Flexible

Now, this REF concept can be and should be planned into your nutrition program. Let us elaborate:

R - Realistic: You need to have a nutrition program that's realistic for your goals, lifestyle, schedule, etc

E - Enjoyable: You need to have a nutrition program that's enjoyable because if you hate the nutrition programs then you aren't going to be adherent and consistent, which is the number one factor in attaining results.

F - Flexible: You need to have a nutrition program that's flexible because let's say you follow a rigid meal plan and something

---

[16] "Muscle and Strength Training Pyramid Level 1 and intro - YouTube." 2015. <https://www.youtube.com/watch?v=OWmchPCyDvw>

comes up during the day so you can't have that exact meal, well now you need to be flexible, adapt, and be able to make a good alternate choice to replace that meal.

If you consider REF into your nutrition program, we can almost guarantee that adherence and consistency will be elevated and thus more results will be attained.

Advanced Stage:

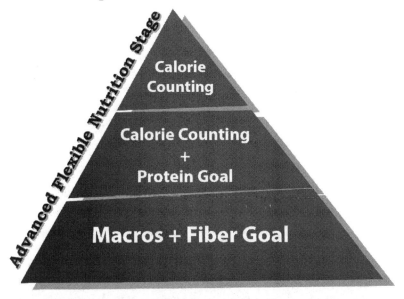

Advanced Flexible Nutrition Stage

Calorie Counting

Calorie Counting
+
Protein Goal

Macros + Fiber Goal

dynamicduotraining.com

The moment everyone has been waiting for is finally here and that's to have reached the advanced level within nutrition. Once you have reached the advanced level, you will have some more tools in your tool box from going through the beginner and intermediate levels, and that our friends, will allow you to have flexibility and long-term sustainability within your nutrition program.

If you mastered the intermediate principles, then you should follow the advanced nutrition recommendations below:

Calorie Counting

The research is very clear on calorie counting, and it demonstrates that calorie counting is beneficial. In a study by Wadden and colleagues, it showed people who frequently recorded their food intake lost over twice as much weight as people who infrequently recorded their food intake.[17]

Baker and colleagues showed that self-monitoring of food intake was positively associated with weight loss success, and not monitoring at all was negatively associated with weight change.[18]

This doesn't mean you have to count calories to be successful. However, the research shows that you are more likely to be successful if you do. Again, it's just an awareness tool. It is something we advocate if you are looking to take your physique to the next level.

Calorie Counting with a Protein Goal

We just hit on why calorie counting is important and something we recommend if you want to enhance your physique. Let's say you really want to optimize your physique. Well, now you may want to set a protein goal because from a physique enhancement standpoint,

---

[17]   Wadden, Thomas A et al. "Randomized trial of lifestyle modification and pharmacotherapy for obesity." *New England Journal of Medicine* 353.20 (2005): 2111-2120.

[18]   Baker, Raymond C, and Daniel S Kirschenbaum. "Self-monitoring may be necessary for successful weight control." *Behavior Therapy* 24.3 (1993): 377-394.

protein is a very crucial macronutrient. Plus, here are some other benefits on why you want to have a protein goal:[19]

- Retain or gain muscle mass
- It's the most filling macronutrient over carbohydrates and fats
- Your body works the hardest breaking this nutrient down as opposed to carbs and fats
- Keeps metabolic rate high during dieting since you are retaining muscle mass

As you can see, putting protein at the forefront because of its benefits and then focusing on counting your calories can be a game changer as far as flexibility. We've experimented with this tool a lot on vacations, traveling for business, offseason goals, etc. This has also worked extremely well with clients because of the flexibility of not having to focus on hitting specific carbohydrate and fat goals. So this has really given us good reasons to go with this tool and recommend it to you.

Macronutrients

Okay let's chat macronutrients. Macronutrients are what forms calories through protein, carbohydrates, and fats.[20] We will break down each macronutrient and explain why each has a pivotal role in your nutrition program.

---

19   Moore, Daniel R et al. "Beyond muscle hypertrophy: why dietary protein is important for endurance athletes 1." *Applied Physiology, Nutrition, and Metabolism* 39.9 (2014): 987-997.
20   Whitney E, Rolfes S. Understanding Nutrition. 13th edition. 2013

Protein

Proteins are essential nutritionally because of their basic amino acids, which the body must have to synthesize its own variety of proteins & nitrogen-containing molecules that make life possible. Amino acids are the building blocks of proteins, there are 20 amino acids in the body (9 essential & 11 non-essential) we produce the 9 essential amino acids through food and supplementation and as for the 11 non-essential amino acids, we produce in our bodies by ourselves.

Proteins are the building blocks for muscle tissue. When you work out a muscle group, the muscle tissue is being broken down by the load (weights) and in order to grow and recover, the muscles must be fed amino acids and protein. Protein should be consumed at each of your meals throughout the day.

Carbohydrates

When carbs have been ingested, they are absorbed into the mouth, stomach & intestines to the smaller unit which is usually glucose (blood sugar). The main purpose of carbohydrates is to provide energy and fuel for the body, speed up the body's metabolism to prevent unwanted fat storage & spare muscle protein. Everybody metabolizes Carbs differently. Some people can consume a lot of carbs and stay lean and some just simply can't eat a lot because after their metabolism utilizes a certain amount, the rest will be stored into fat cells. There are 2 different types of carbs: Complex & simple, and it is important to find out which types tailor your body best and how much.

Fats

Fats are the most energy-dense macronutrient & they provide many of the body's tissues & organs with most of their energy. Fats are also essential for building muscle, reducing cortisol levels, providing energy, helps with hunger pains, and assisting the body in functioning properly. Fats also have the most calories per gram out of the macronutrients.

Fiber

Fiber is a part of the carbohydrate family and is very important for the following reasons:

- Fiber tends to sit longer in your GI (Gastrointestinal) which pulls fluids into the area. That's a good thing normally because it makes you feel fuller. A carbohydrate in less fiber will be digested more rapidly and not pull water in your GI like something heavier would with a lot of fiber.
- It is important for gut health and digestive health. If you don't have a healthy digestive system then you aren't going to get good assimilation of nutrients
- It increases thermogenesis and thus helps with fat loss

Once you've decided your personal fitness goals, you can now start counting your macronutrients (daily protein, carbs, and fats) along with hitting a fiber goal which can easily be achieved through eating whole and minimally refined food sources along with a couple servings of fruits and veggies per day.

By counting your daily macronutrients, this will allow you to have more flexibility within your diet. Having more flexibility allows you to eat the foods you like in moderation, not have you eliminate food groups, and still get results. Flexible nutrition has shown a stronger association with lower body weight and the absence of depression and anxiety within a nutrition program.[21] [22]

Moreover, Westenhoefer and colleagues compared rigid control and flexible control eating.[23] [24]

Rigid control is characterized by a dichotomous, all or nothing approach to eating, dieting and weight, aka cookie cutter diet or set meal plan.

Flexible control is characterized by a more gradual approach to eating, dieting, and weight, in which "fattening" foods are eaten in limited quantities without feelings of guilt, aka flexible nutrition.

As you can see, a very rigid diet such as a meal plan or cookie cutter diet where you're either on the diet or off can lead to a lot of problems. This is not a sustainable diet, this will teach you nothing about nutrition or your body, and it will cause problems with schedules, work, family, kids, vacations, and activities.

The caveat to flexible nutrition is one can be too "flexible" and get away from some of the basics they learned in the beginners level; hence the majority of the diet should comprise of high quality food sources. But this needs to be trialed through self-experimentation.

[21]   Stewart, Tiffany M, Donald A Williamson, and Marney A White. "Rigid vs. flexible dieting: association with eating disorder symptoms in nonobese women." *Appetite* 38.1 (2002): 39-44.

[22]   Smith, CF et al. "Flexible vs. Rigid dieting strategies: relationship with adverse behavioral outcomes." *Appetite* 32.3 (1999): 295-305.

[23]   Westenhoefer, Joachim, Albert J Stunkard, and Volker Pudel. "Validation of the flexible and rigid control dimensions of dietary restraint." *International Journal of Eating Disorders* 26.1 (1999): 53-64.

[24]   Westenhoefer, Joachim et al. "Cognitive and weight-related correlates of flexible and rigid restrained eating behaviour." *Eating behaviors* 14.1 (2013): 69-72.

Hierarchy of Flexible Nutrition

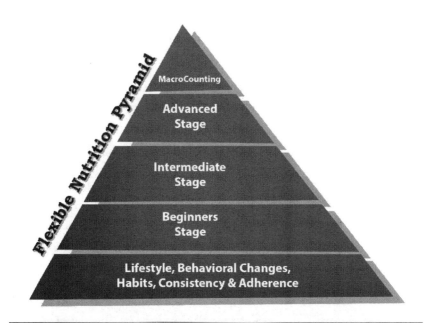

Now that you have a good understanding of what flexible nutrition looks like through a beginner, intermediate, and advanced stages, we want to present to you a hierarchy of flexible nutrition.

Feel free to take a picture of the infographic above or hell, even cut it out and paste it on your fridge.

We don't want this to be looked at as another quick fix dieting book or system, because it's absolutely not that. While research shows that being ambitious with goals correlates with improved outcomes,[25] we

---

[25] Stice, Eric. "Risk and maintenance factors for eating pathology: a meta-analytic review." *Psychological bulletin* 128.5 (2002): 825.

also know rigidity and restrictions can begin a vicious dieting cycle where the individual restricts excessively, deprivation, and counter-regulatory mechanisms are activated, not to mention disinhibition and a lapse in dietary compliance.[26] Post failure attempts to restrict become even more vigorous and strict.

What's great about the above pyramid we have created is it's a nice guide for whenever you want to step it up a notch and enhance your physique, so you simply go into the advanced stage level and above and get to work until you achieve your physique goals.

On the contrary, say life throws you a curveball, your stress is high, sleep is off, and just plain craziness. Well, you taper down the bottom of the pyramid and just go back to the fundamentals within nutrition until life is less overwhelming.

The key to long-term sustainability isn't in perfection or restriction, it's in mastering the art of getting through periods of stress, fatigue, chaos, lack of motivation, and unexpected events both big and small - the unpredictability that is life.[27]

Don't get us wrong here, it will take some practice and self-experimentation on when to back off rigidity and when you need to push through and find alternatives. This is where a good experienced and rationale trainer/coach comes into play. They will be your objective and unbiased eye.

The main goal is to promote maximal flexibility while actively progressing towards a goal - whether it be general improved health and wellness, fat loss, contest prep, or just wanting to look great naked.

Overall, as we've stated many times throughout this chapter, adherence and consistency is king to whatever any diet book or new fad diet claims.

---

[26]   Hill, Andrew J. "Does dieting make you fat?." *British Journal of Nutrition* 92.S1 (2004): S15-S18.

[27]   Linde, Jennifer A et al. "Are unrealistic weight loss goals associated with outcomes for overweight women?." *Obesity Research* 12.3 (2004): 569-576.

Flexible nutrition is a continuum, not an on or off switch. There's nothing wrong with going from the very bottom of this pyramid up to the very peak of it, slowly, and gradually. On the contrary, there's nothing wrong with being at the top of the pyramid after working to get there and you're there for "x" amount of months and then all of a sudden you want to spend some time in the middle of the pyramid or the bottom. It's flexible and it should be tailored to your goals, schedule, personal preferences, times of the year, and what you can realistically stick to for days, weeks, months and years. Use the pyramid as a guide and enjoy being flexible with your nutrition.

Dynamic Tips

- Consistency, adherence, and habits will trump any diet that's out there. You must see yourself on a diet for days, weeks, months, and years so it can become a lifestyle.
- Focus on building a strong foundation within your nutrition program by learning the basics in the beginner's stage.
- Slowly advance through the nutrition stages and don't be afraid to go back to the stages to build momentum, increase consistency and adherence, and thus reap the results.

Do you want to learn more about Flexible Nutrition?
We have some game changing exercises in our Dynamic Lifestyle workbook for you. To get the workbook and enter The New Era of Fitness, go to
www.TheNewEraOfFitness.com/bonus

CHAPTER 7

Flexible Exercise

"Fitness is not about being better than someone else.
It's about being better than you used to be."

– Brett Hoebel

Just like we discussed in the last chapter with flexible nutrition, the fitness industry is full of bad exercise programming and gimmicky workouts that promise you this and that when it comes to results.

Instead of giving you a cookie cutter workout program, we want to teach you principles, tools, and training methodology that's been around for a long time and will take you much further than the "next best workout" or gimmicky exercises that promise muscle growth and strength with five pound pink dumbbells.

We know this doesn't sound sexy, but we care more about helping you get results.

The Flexible exercise pyramid we have created below will help guide you on your exercise journey. You will build solid training principles, you will have more tools in your belt, and the training methodology will get you results over time.

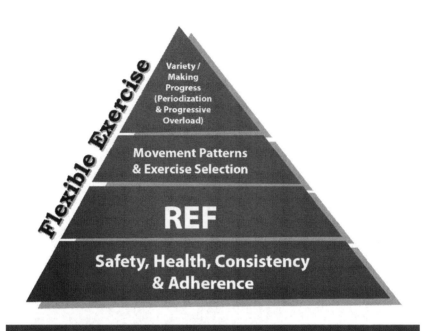

Flexible Exercise

Variety /
Making
Progress
(Periodization
& Progressive
Overload)

Movement Patterns
& Exercise Selection

REF

Safety, Health, Consistency
& Adherence

dynamicduotraining.com

The 4 Most Underrated Factors in Exercise

Many are surprised to learn that they are consistency, adherence, safety, and health?

Just think about this for a second, and you'll see why these are underrated...

Using safety in your exercises leads to staying healthy.

Staying healthy leads to adherence and consistency.

Adherence and consistency within exercise leads to results.

We can't advocate the importance of adherence and consistency enough when it comes to your fitness journey. Trust us, we know it's hard to not sometimes want to take that quick and easy elevator to get our end results, but trust us again when we say, it's that much sweeter learning to appreciate the process and building those habits to achieve adherence and consistency.

A 2012 study by Fishbach and Choi studied two groups. One group focused all its attention specifically on the end goal related to performing the selected task, and the other group focused on the process of performing the task itself. The first group was instructed to try to self-motivate by focusing on what they would eventually achieve by doing the task, while the second group was instructed to focus on the positive feelings they had while performing the task. The results showed the group that focused on the end goal, rather than the process, actually achieved their goals with less consistency.[28]

This is a fascinating study because we can easily apply this to fitness. The first group would focus on setting new PBs or PRs (personal bests or personal records) on squats, bench, deadlifts, or any exercise; the second group would focus on how the acts of these exercises make you feel strong, unstoppable, and productive. The study we just spoke about goes to show that you need to enjoy the process instead of having the mindset of just achieving the end goal...this will lead to more adherence and enjoyment over your fitness journey.

Make sure to use safety when training; proper form is always advocated. Make sure to stay healthy so you can progress and not be on the sidelines. Make sure to enjoy the process to increase adherence and consistency so you can attain your desired results.

---

[28] Fishbach, Ayelet, and Jinhee Choi. "When thinking about goals undermines goal pursuit." *Organizational Behavior and Human Decision Processes* 118.2 (2012): 99-107.

Being REF'd Up

If only we could travel back in time and know what we know now, maybe we would be world-class powerlifters or competing at the Olympics…In our wildest dreams!

All joking aside, we remember following cookie cutter training programs out of muscle magazines, copying trainers' workouts at gyms, following workouts out of books, basically doing whatever we could to grow muscle and get strong.

Our efforts and desires were great, but the main issues were that we were too rigid with our training, thought in black and white terms, thought there were yes and no answers, didn't apply context, didn't focus on training quality, and weren't 100% in-tune with our bodies. Not to mention, we weren't being REF'd up enough. You are probably saying to yourself, what the hell does REF'd up mean in the context of exercise?

Being REF'd up simply means using REF within an exercise program.[29]

R - Realistic: Exercise program needs to be realistic for your schedule and goals

E - Enjoyable: Exercise program needs to be enjoyable to work harder at

F - Flexible: Exercise program needs to be flexible in case life factors occur

---

[29] Eric Helms. The muscle and strength pyramid training. 2016

Examples of Why You Need REF within Your Exercise

Being Realistic with Exercise:

> Monday rolls around, you have your weekly training outlined, your workout spreadsheet says you're training 5 days this week, but out of nowhere your boss wants you to take on a last minute project, and they need you to fly out of town tomorrow morning.

> First reaction is… "That SOB!"

> The second reaction is, "Now what do I do with my training week that's already outlined and how will I complete 5 training days?"

> The answer is that there is not much you can do besides adapt and be realistic about the situation. Just looking at this scenario, do you really think your training week is going to go 100% accordingly to plan now?

> Probably not, so you need to be realistic about what kind of exercise program you can achieve due to your goals, schedule, time constraints, family, etc.

Enjoyment within Exercise:

> It's time to head to your weekly Pilates class, but you're dragging your feet. You thought it sounded interesting, but you aren't really enjoying the class. It's boring and you just can't get excited about it. You finally convince yourself to go, but you don't get much out of the class.

> Do you think you are actually going to stick to that workout and benefit from it? Probably not. Chances are, you'll start coming up with reasons to ditch the class to do something you actually enjoy.

Find/create a workout plan that motivates and excites you. You should want to show up to classes or the gym.

On the other hand, if you just focus on enjoyment into your training, do you think your training program will be "optimal?" Do you think you're really going to challenge yourself?

Probably not and here's why, say you enjoy circuit style training and your goal is to build maximum strength and optimize muscle growth, and you end up programming your entire training protocol around circuit style training.

We can almost guarantee that your strength on the main lifts (squat, bench press, deadlift, overhead press, and rowing variations) will be hindered from the shorter rest periods and fatigue that circuit training produces. Thus, how will you maximize progressive overload? This has been shown to be one of the major factors in inducing maximum muscle growth and strength.[30]

Same thing for someone who loves to do the 3 main lifts (squats, bench press, deadlift). Say this person wants to do these 3 main lifts 4-5 days per week at high intensities (because they love to train heavy and grunt), we highly doubt they will recover from this frequency and intensity (amount of training days and heavy lifting) and they may even regress from not completing all of the work or will end up getting injured.[31]

The main point is you need balance; you absolutely need to enjoy your program to train harder at it and thus get results;

---

[30]   Fleck 2004; Stone 2007
[31]   Gillam 1981; Stone 1987

however, you also need to know what's "optimal" for your goals, challenge yourself by trying new workouts or programs, and sometimes that requires not doing some of those things you truly enjoy most of the time because that could lead to mediocrity and complacency.

Being Flexible within Exercise:

When you apply flexibility into your programming, it opens a lot of doors. This allows you to complete your total training volume (reps x sets x load) over the course of a week. This has been proven to be one of the biggest factors in increasing muscle mass and strength.[32]

Let's say you have four main lifts planned (Squats, Dumbbell bench press, Barbell overhead presses, Barbell hip thrusts) and 3 secondary lifts planned (Back extensions, Lateral raises, Lunges). Well, what if these 2 things occurred?

1. You know you have to complete these 7 workouts on Tuesday; that's what your program says and your coach or trainer says, "You just have to do it, no ifs or buts about it." But you found out that you have to go back to the office to work and you only have 45 minutes to train. Odds are you won't complete these 7 workouts in a productive manner in 45 minutes. So, the flexibility part comes in; you can remove the secondary lifts and do them later in the week.

2. Say after the four main lifts, your shoulders and quads are fried. It's just one of those days when those 4 lifts kicked your ass, sleep wasn't great the night before, and stress was

---

[32] Schoenfeld 2014; Flann 2011; Goto 2004

high in the morning, but you still have 3 secondary lifts to complete. Odds are the lateral raises and lunges are going to kick your ass more, which may lead to doing less weight or reps, more soreness that will affect the next day's training, and thus, less overall volume. So maybe you leave the lateral raises for later in the week and replace seated leg extensions for lunges that day.

Flexibility in training is a beautiful thing, so long as you:

- Complete your total training volume (reps x sets x load) over the course of a week and in easier terms just make sure to get all your workouts done over the course of a week
- Sequence and order your main and secondary lifts correctly. Make sure to do your compound-multi joint exercises first followed by your smaller-single joint exercises. You'll learn more about this later in the chapter.
- Include proper exercise selection to induce workout quality, reduce soreness, and burnout. It's important to choose exercises that are suitable for your body type, leverages, anatomy, biomechanics, etc.
- Making sure you're still progressing properly. You want to make sure you're adding reps, sets, exercises, weight overtime throughout your training career. See more info below.

If you consider adding REF into your training programming, we promise that your weekly training sessions will be planned better and your daily training sessions will be more productive, and this will lead to more results.

Become a Master at these Movement Patterns

"I fear not the man who has practiced 10,000 kicks once, but I fear the man who has practiced one kick 10,000 times."

– Bruce Lee

We know that theory, applied science, and actual application are all needed in fitness. Research studies are the theory, books based on studies are the applied science, and then actually training-coaching clients and writing programs is the application.

Through all three of these, we have found that there are four basic movement patterns a beginner needs to learn in order to teach their brains to become more efficient and thus continue to progress over time, whether that's adding more volume, adding more frequency, increasing intensity, doing more advanced exercises, or a combination of all.[33]

With these basic movement patterns, we want you to think like Bruce Lee did and practice these over and over, so you eventually master them.

The four basic movement patterns you want to learn are:

Push Exercise:

- Overhead Barbell/Dumbbell Press
- Barbell/Dumbbell Bench Press (Recommended)
- Barbell/Dumbbell Floor Press

---

[33]   Mark Rippetoe and Andy Baker. Practical programming for strength training. 2013

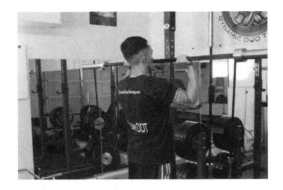

Pull Exercise:

- Bent over Barbell/Dumbbell Rows
- Chin Up, Pull Up or Pulldown (Recommended)
- Seated Cable Row
- Standing T Bar Row

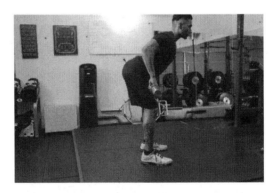

Squat/Lunge Exercise:

- Barbell Squat (Recommended)
- Front Squat
- Box Squat
- Leg Press/Hack Squat
- Lunges

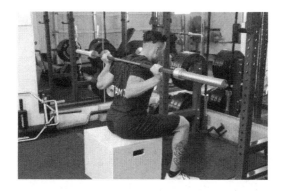

Hip Hinge Exercise:

- Deadlift (Recommended)
- Barbell Glute Bridge/Barbell Hip Thrusts
- RDL's

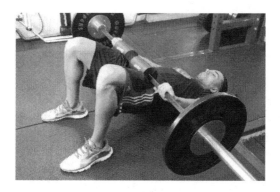

If you master these four basic movement patterns, 99.9% of the time, you will be able to progress more efficiently and set yourself up for proper training habits, long-term progress, and athletic achievement.

Exercise Selection to Increase Strength

The importance of exercise selection varies depending on perspective, but in the context of a beginner-intermediate, it's important to take into consideration and emphasize choosing proper exercises to increase strength.

In Eric Helms' *Muscle and Strength Pyramid Training*, he states:

For hypertrophy (muscle growth), a wide variety of exercises can be used to stimulate growth. That being said, based on the biomechanics of the individual, some exercises may be more effective than others. This is also relevant consideration for a strength athlete. For example, even though a powerlifter may have to squat, in some cases the squat may not produce balanced development if that specific powerlifter is not well built to squat. Therefore they might be better suited to doing more assistance work for leg development rather than more squats compared to someone who had limb and torso lengths well suited to squatting.

Another important aspect we need to consider is that exercise selection should be centered on the goal of your training, that means whether you're training purely for muscle mass like a bodybuilder or training for strength like a powerlifter.

We recommend a beginner-intermediate starts with multi-joint or compound movements like the four exercises we suggested above and then focus on secondary or isolation exercises.

It's important to properly order your exercises in a manner where you can:[34][35]

[34] "Essentials of Strength Training and Conditioning-3rd Edition." 2008.
<http://nirsa.humankinetics.com/showproduct.cfm?isbn=9780736058032>
[35] Zatsiorsky, Vladimir M, and William J Kraemer. *Science and practice of strength training*. Human Kinetics, 2006.

- Put enough effort into each rep, and perform that rep correctly
- Put enough effort into each set
- Select the right exercises and order them effectively within the training session
- Make sure the session accomplished its purpose
- Make sure the training week itself is laid out well to allow yourself to train hard within each session and recover effectively between sessions so you can progress

Having Variety in Your Exercise and Constantly Making Progress

"The question shouldn't be does it work? The question should be is it optimal?"

As the words left the respected Dr. Mike Zourdos mouth, we looked at each other with our caterpillar eyebrows raised high as if we had the same exact thought.

Sitting at the 2014 NSCA conference in July, we had listened to lots of incredible speakers and some of the greatest minds in the industry.

But for the last year, we had really been focusing on specializing training programs for different programming. It was this one line that best summarized our most recent approach.

This stuck with us because there is no such thing as optimal, but when you seek for something to be optimal, it creates discussion, brings questioning, theories, and thus leads to studies being conducted. So every time we put a client's training program together, we ask, "Is this going to be optimal?"

Designing a training program isn't rocket science, but it's still a science and there should be some intelligent programming involved using training methodology and exercise science. There's a reason why certain people get better results than others. We are going to tell you some ways to build an optimal training program so that you can be one of those outliers getting great results.

Use Periodization

Not to get too technical on periodization because we can write an entire book on this, but just remember this:

"Non-periodization" means no variation

"Periodization" means variation

The key factor involved in going towards an individual's potential is 'variation' in exercise stimulus with systematic rest, volume, intensity, frequency, and exercise selection programmed into the equation.[36][37]

Once you know that you want to incorporate periodization into your training and have variety, you then need to figure out what concept you want to use. There are various concepts within periodization, such as:

- Linear periodization
- Non-linear periodization
- Daily/Weekly undulated periodization
- Auto-regulated training/RPE

Once you have the concept you want to use, you then need to program the length of how long you will be training under this concept:

---

[36] Bompa and Haff. Periodization: Theory and methodology of training 5th edition. 2009
[37] Stone, Michael H et al. "A Theoretical Model of Strength Training." *Strength & Conditioning Journal* 4.4 (1982): 36-39.

- Microcycles → Weeks to 1 month
- Mesocycles → Month to months
- Macrocycles → Months to a year

Now that you have your cycles figured out, you will need to use training variables, such as:[38]

- Intensity → % of 1 Repetition Maximum
- Frequency → How many days a week you will be training and each body part
- Volume → Total work output, sets x reps x weight

Now that you have your training variables incorporated, you can start reaping the benefits of increasing strength, building muscle mass, and looking and feeling great.

Use the Three Mechanisms of Hypertrophy

With hypertrophy (muscle growth), you need periodization (variety), and you need to dig a little deeper within your training programming to get there.

Brad Schoenfeld found that there are three mechanisms to muscle growth and those are:[39]

- Mechanical tension
- Muscle damage
- Metabolic stress/Cell swelling

---

[38] Wernbom, Mathias, Jesper Augustsson, and Roland Thomeé. "The influence of frequency, intensity, volume and mode of strength training on whole muscle cross-sectional area in humans." *Sports medicine* 37.3 (2007): 225-264.

[39] Schoenfeld, Brad J. "The mechanisms of muscle hypertrophy and their application to resistance training." *The Journal of Strength & Conditioning Research* 24.10 (2010): 2857-2872.

Mechanical tension relates to how long the muscle is under tension, so heavy loads would be your best bet here.

Muscle damage relates to localized damage to muscle tissue, which leads to more of a growth response in muscle, so moderate loads and exercises that stretch the muscle more, like lunges or RDLs, would be your best bet here.

Metabolic stress relates to metabolite accumulation through lactate, hydrogen ions, creatine, etc. So light loads are your best bet here.

When we put this all together, we have repetition ranges that could vary from 1-30 reps and should be properly used and programmed intelligently into a training program.

Increase your Volume over Time

Remember that volume is reps x sets x load lifted. For example, you do squats for 3 sets of 6 reps at 225 lbs, the total volume is 4,050 lbs.

Volume has been shown to be one of the most important training variables in inducing muscle growth and strength.[40][41]

Alterations of training load and volume have been shown to affect hormonal, neural, and hypertrophic responses and continuous adaptations to resistance training.[42] Tan and colleagues suggest that the interplay between load and volume is the critical factor in determining the optimal range of training stimuli in order to promote the neuromuscular adaptations associated with resistance training.[43]

---

[40] Krieger, James W. "Single vs. multiple sets of resistance exercise for muscle hypertrophy: a meta-analysis." *The Journal of Strength & Conditioning Research* 24.4 (2010): 1150-1159.

[41] Krieger, James W. "Single versus multiple sets of resistance exercise: a meta-regression." *The Journal of Strength & Conditioning Research* 23.6 (2009): 1890-1901.

[42] Bird, Stephen P, Kyle M Tarpenning, and Frank E Marino. "Designing resistance training programmes to enhance muscular fitness." *Sports medicine* 35.10 (2005): 841-851.

[43] Tan, Benedict. "Manipulating Resistance Training Program Variables to Optimize Maximum Strength in Men: A Review." *The Journal of Strength & Conditioning Research* 13.3 (1999): 289-304.

Think of volume like dieting, you want to diet on as many calories as you can, and when your weight stagnates, you want to progress appropriately and not cut 1,000 calories, maybe cut 200 calories and lose at a modest pace. Same thing with training volume. If you plateau, you shouldn't add in a ton of volume, maybe add in a little more and progress appropriately over time.

Don't be a Program Hopper

One of our biggest pet peeves in the gym is seeing "program hopping." Program hopping is a huge problem in one's training arsenal. Most people at various points in their training careers lose sight of the basis for all productive training. They forget that the goal is always to produce a stress that induces adaptation through recovery and supercompensation.

Variety for variety's sake is pointless. All training must be planned, and success must be planned for it. If you have good success with an exercise program thus far, then change for the sake of change itself makes no sense. In fact, staying within this program longer means the possibility of more subtle alterations, which in turn means less risk of losing valuable training time through trial and error process that accompanies major overhauls in programming.

Training is a skill, and you need time to practice exercises to get good at them and progress properly so you can get stronger and thus add more muscle mass. Too many times, we see people jumping from Crossfit to Insanity to bodybuilding to bodyweight training... the list can go on. Stick to one form of training for 4-16 weeks and progress appropriately.

Keep a Training Log to Track Your Data and Keep Progressing

As Big Ben Franklin said, "Failing to plan is planning to fail."

This may have to be second on the list of gym pet peeves - when someone doesn't track their training progress in a training log at the gym and just goes through the motions.

→ A training log is kept by every serious trainee as a record of his or her training progress. It is a crucial source of data for determinations such as:

☐ Staleness

☐ Overtraining

☐ Effectiveness of newly added exercises

☐ Tracking volume

☐ Effectiveness of overall training protocol

→ Constantly making progress with progressive overload

It's absolutely crucial to keep ensuring progressive overload during your training career.

What does this mean?

It means to have some sort of progression such as adding weight, adding reps, adding sets, adding exercises, etc. If your main goal is putting on muscle, focus more on progressions that increase volume, and if your main goal is strength, focus more on progressions that increase load (amount of weight lifted).

Another form of tracking we've been experimenting with is "informal note taking" during our training.

This is a great way to:

- Gage your effort during sets when not lifting to muscular failure
- Help with the planning of your training
- Help reduce the tendency to train to failure on every set of every exercise
- Keep you healthy and more fresh for your workouts for more quality workouts
- Be more in tuned with your body
- Have you increasing your training volume over time

There's some good data supporting this.[44][45] Try using informal note taking on the main lifts like this:

- Feelings like: "easy," "medium," or "hard"
- Use a 5 point scale where 1 is easy and 5 is hard
- Use the RIR scale (repetitions in reserve scale of 7-10) 7 being you had 3 reps left in the tank, 8 being you had 2 reps left in the tank, 9 being 1 rep left in the tank, and 10 being you had no reps left in the tank and it was maximum failure.

These informal notes and training log records helps us look back at our training and forces us to pay attention to it more, helps us assign and adjust load and volume depending on environmental and lifestyle factors, helps us reflect on and honestly evaluate each set, and helps keep our working sets dialed into that zone of quality.

Just ask yourself this question, "Would you go on a road trip without a road map?" So why go into the gym without a plan?

---

[44] "Publications for Daniel Hackett 2016 2015 2014 2013 2012." 2015. <https://sydney.edu.au/health-sciences/about/people/publications/daniel.hackett.pdf>/ Hackette. The Journal of Sports Sciences. 2012

[45] Zourdos, Michael C, Marcos A Sanchez-Gonzalez, and Sara E Mahoney. "A brief review: the implications of iron supplementation for marathon runners on health and performance." *The Journal of Strength & Conditioning Research* 29.2 (2015): 559-565.

Success and Peaks and Valleys within Exercise

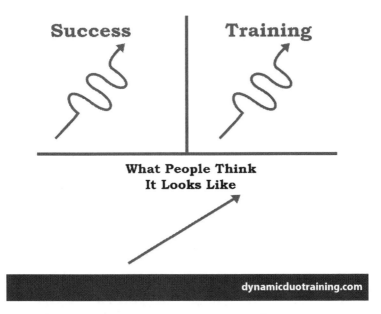

When you hear the word "success," who is the first person that comes to mind? Now, if you could ask that person if their success came in a straight line or had ups and downs, we can almost guarantee 99.9% that it had ups and downs. Same with exercise; think of an inspiring person whose physique you would want. To attain that physique it took years, hard work, consistency, and a lot of peaks and valleys.

You are going to go through peaks and valleys in your training, but the main premise should be that your peaks are exceeding your older peaks and your valleys are exceeding your older valleys.

This way you are slowly, but surely ensuring progress within your training.

Not a lot of people want to put up with this slow and hard grind within training to ensure progress and get results.

We find that too many people look at their training blocks (could be anywhere from 4-20 weeks) in a microscope. They expect to put on 50 lbs on their squats, bench, and deadlifts after each training block (150 total pounds). Just really think about it. That means someone would potentially put on approximately 390-1,950 total pounds to their main lifts each year and that would lead to adding a ton of muscle and strength year in and year out, That's just not realistic and it doesn't work like that.

Another form of impatience we see is this:

Have you ever been pissed at yourself for not completing that last rep or perhaps skipping that last set because you just weren't feeling it that day?

This goes in hand with any periodization model. Don't get so wrapped up in one down day or performance. For example, you plan on hitting 3 sets of squats for 8 reps at a specific load, and on the third set you come up 2 reps short. Don't let this ruin your day; it's one day of fluctuation in the grand scheme of things. There will always be another day.

One down day or performance isn't going to impede your strength or muscle growth gains. Look at the big picture of the training block or program and just be prepared to do your job the next training day.

Creating the Best Program

Training must be periodized and it must have enough volume to stimulate growth. Contrary to what most people believe, volume, intensity, frequency, muscle damage, mechanical load, metabolic stress, power, and strength are all important for muscle growth; however volume seems to be the most important based on the research.[46][47]

[46]   Krieger, JW. Single vs multiple sets of resistance training exercise. 2009
[47]   Krieger, JW. Single vs multiple sets of resistance training exercise for muscle hypertrophy. 2010

What does it all mean? You have two options:

1. Keep studying and digging deeper into each of these areas that help you build the best workout possible for your body and your goals. We've been studying this material for 10 years now, and we still continue to learn. After working with over a thousand clients, it's allowed us to have a better idea of not only how to create programs, but also how to adjust them as needed. Your job is then to learn about one at a time, and then apply that knowledge to your own programs.

2. Find a coach/trainer and let them take care of the programming for you—but always be sure to ask questions. All great coaches look towards other coaches to help them look and feel their best. When we did our bodybuilding shows, we hired a coach. When our mentors prepare for the stage, they hire a coach. Why? Because putting your health in the hands of someone with an outside perspective is the best way to remove any bias and directly attack all your weaknesses.

Now get out there, use these concepts and principles we have taught you, train hard, be smart, be consistent, and have fun!

Dynamic Tips

- Safety, health, consistency, and adherence will override any magical, overpromised or "next best" exercise program.
- Include REF (Realistic, Enjoyable, and Flexible) in your exercise program for more consistency, adherence, and results.
- Slowly advance through your exercise program by adding volume over your training career, make sure you're doing

some sort of progressive overload, and understand there will be peaks and valleys throughout your training journey and that's perfectly okay.

Do you want to learn more about Dynamic Fitness?
We have some game changing exercises in our Dynamic Lifestyle workbook for you. To get the workbook and enter The New Era of Fitness, go to
www.TheNewEraOfFitness.com/bonus

CHAPTER 8

Four Pillars of Life

"Life isn't about finding yourself, it's about creating yourself."
– George Bernard Shaw

Our mentor, Tai Lopez, of Tailopez.com, once said, "In order to live the Good Life, you have to constantly pay attention and balance out the Four Pillars of Life." Each area of our lives must be treated with the type of respect, love, care and focus that we put in others. If you are not familiar with the Four Pillars of Life, they are as follows:

- Health
- Wealth
- Love
- Happiness

Unfortunately, many people overlook these four pillars. Think about how busy we all get with our days and responsibilities. Work, school, family, kids, stress, gym, the list goes on and on. If you take a second to just look at those four pillars of life above, you will understand that those are the pillars that make life beautiful. If you can say that all of those pillars are fulfilled in your life, you must be living the good life and have nothing to worry about. For the majority of society, this will make or break them from going forward in life and possibly cause a lot of problems.

89

We are guilty ourselves and never really paid any attention to these pillars of life. Thinking back on it now, no wonder we were in such a dark place, full of pain, anger and just overall lost with life. If we would have discovered these four pillars of life earlier on and really made the effort to pay attention and improve in each area, we could have been much happier individuals in our youth.

If you have dealt with losses in your family, we are sure you can agree with us that health, wealth, love, and happiness are non-existent for quite some time. We experienced this and we want to save you from experiencing the same thing. If something bad ever happens in your life, revert back to these four pillars as fast as you can and focus on what you can control. Let's look into these four pillars more in depth now.

• Health

Let's face it, without your overall health, you cannot enjoy or master the other pillars of life. Health overrules everything. Think about how many wealthy, intelligent, and successful people there are around the world who do not take care of their overall health. Often times, we get so consumed with what is in front of us that we put our health on the back burner. We have supplied you with a very generous amount of information regarding nutrition and training in the previous chapters, so stop procrastinating and take action already on your health! Develop that crystal clear vision!

You might be saying, "Well, you guys are health advocates and have to maintain your overall health and have to lead by example." That is very true, but on the flip side, if we didn't take care of our overall health, we wouldn't be able to do what we love and find the energy to get wealthier, we wouldn't be able to find a significant other to love or even have self-love for ourselves, and we damn sure wouldn't be happy. We are not saying you have to look like a fitness model, just start with 30 minutes per day and focus on your overall health, then build upon that as time goes on. No matter what anyone says, your overall health should be at the top of your priority list now and for the long haul. You cannot be productive if you are constantly in and out of the hospital battling your health.

• Wealth

The word wealth means several different things to us, such as: having more money, more power, success, traveling, changing lives, and leaving a legacy. What is your first thought when you see or hear the word wealth? We ask you this question because you should have your own definition of the word wealth. Once you figure out what your definition is, write it out and put it somewhere visible. You can also rate yourself from 1 to 10 for your current wealth and ask yourself, "What choices can I make today to set myself up for long-term financial freedom?"

Let's take a moment and use some of our definitions for wealth that we listed above. Everything we listed is what gets us motivated every day to be the best versions of ourselves and get 1% better all around. One in particular, traveling, really gets us excited! We love the thought of being able to get up and travel anywhere we want at any point in time. This is wealth to us! Once you find out what you see as wealth, it will help motivate you even more and make you want to attain that goal or dream. Keep in mind, without your health, you cannot enjoy your wealth.

• Love

You don't need to talk to someone with a PhD to understand love. Ask your grandma what her definition of love is. We guarantee, her answer will make you light up like a Christmas tree. Maybe some of us are not looking to be in love with a significant other right at the moment, but eventually you would like to experience it and ultimately think it's the key to being happy. Maybe some of us are looking for love within families and friendships first. Everyone is looking for something different when it comes to love, it really comes down to where they are in their life.

We feel the majority of people need to be looking to improve their self-love before anything. Self-love is so overlooked in today's society. If you were able to give yourself more self-love, ultimately you would be happier with yourself, and it would be a happier world all around.

It comes down to where you are in life and what you are seeking to improve upon. Sure the status quo suggests we all need to fall in love and live happily ever after, right? If only it was that simple and that linear. Love starts with being comfortable with who you are, being vulnerable, knowing your identity, and knowing what your calling is in life. You have to start with self-love and know you are wonderful and loveable inside. Not because others think so. Self-worth comes from only one place, yourself! If you cannot love yourself, how can you expect to fall in love with someone else or show others love? Ask yourself, "How can I give more and allow myself to be vulnerable with the people who really care about me?"

• Happiness

The last and final pillar of life, ladies and gentlemen, is happiness! If you want to be happy, you have to teach your old brain some new tricks and start thinking more optimistically! We live in a world where one little thing can shift our mindsets and completely ruin our train of thought, mood, and day. For instance, many people use their social media to express how "happy" they are or they compare themselves to other people's glamorous lives. This is complete bullshit! There are so many distractions and misleading things in today's society. You cannot get caught up in all that bullshit out there. Think more positive thoughts for yourself first, then worry about another person's happiness.

When you train your brain to think more positive thoughts, you are more likely to form positive habits, which then lead you to more positive results.[48] We know it is not easy to always think positive. Let's face it, life is full of ups and downs. Often during tough down times in life, we find ourselves stuck in a downward "negative-thought spiral." All too quickly, we go from thinking "this one thing sucks" to "my whole day sucks" to "my whole world sucks"!

True happiness is about the thoughts you have, what you have, and who you have in your life. We choose whether or not to enjoy what happens to us. If you take responsibility for everything in your life (including your happiness), you'll find yourself enjoying the little moments and things that truly matter in life.

---

[48] "Happy Brain, Happy Life | Psychology Today." 2015.
<https://www.psychologytoday.com/blog/prime-your-gray-cells/201108/happy-brain-happy-life>

Balancing out all Four Pillars of Life

John Maxwell said, "There's nothing like staring reality in the face to make a person recognize the need for change. Change alone doesn't bring growth but you cannot have growth without change."

Now that you have an understanding of all the Four Pillars of Life, it's time to take action and make some changes in each Pillar of Life. Nobody has this all figured out. These pillars should constantly be changing as time goes on, as you get wiser, or as different life instances happen. The most important thing is to make a change in each area. Do not get complacent with your Pillars of Life. We know we will honor our word and continue to grow in each area, make sure to keep your word and do the same. In your workbook, you will find an exercise to hold you accountable.

Dynamic Tips

- Become familiar with each of the 4 pillars
- Be aware of which one you lack the most currently and take action on it
- Put these 4 pillars somewhere visible so they constantly remind you daily

Ready to focus on the four Pillars of Life?
We have some game changing exercises in our Dynamic Lifestyle workbook for you. To get the workbook and enter The New Era of Fitness, go to
www.TheNewEraOfFitness.com/bonus

Conclusion

A New Era of Fitness is here and you have all the tools you need to create a Dynamic Life filled with health, joy, and prosperity. Remember, fitness is no longer just about going to the gym or focusing on the number on the scale. It is so much more than that! Within your lifestyle, you need to remember the following:

- Create good habits to be successful within fitness.
- Develop good systems around fitness that are going to work with your life, schedule, etc.
- Have a social life around fitness. Anybody that doesn't have a social life is unhappy, whether they admit it or not.
- Balance out work and fitness.
- If you go to school, you need to find time to work out, study, work and go to class.
- Whether you're in a committed relationship or relationships with family or friends, you need to find time for that along with fitness.
- Travel and vacations are needed and a big part of most people's lives, you will need to know how to balance this with fitness.

Within mindset, you need to remember the following:

- You will need to develop a relentless mindset because there will be times where you encounter challenges within fitness and life, whether you get injured and feel like quitting or

95

you fail a diet, go on a binge, and regain the weight back. You will need to be relentless, learn from your mistakes, and march forward.

- If you don't have a crystal clear vision or goals within fitness and lifestyle, the likelihood of you succeeding within your fitness journey won't be as high because motivation will be down.
- Shit is going to happen in life, whether you like it or not, and you will be thrown curveballs, whether it's losing a loved one, going through a breakup or divorce, or losing your job. The question is can you balance fitness and reframe your mindset to look at these curses as blessings and overcome adversity.
- As our good friend, Layne Norton says, "Outwork!" You will need to stay hungry and outwork yourself or your competition, depending on your goals. Once one goal is achieved, you will need to be hungry enough to achieve another one.

Within nutrition, you need to remember the following:

- Consistency, adherence, and habits will trump any diet that's out there. You must see yourself on a diet for days, weeks, months, and years so it can become a lifestyle.
- Focus on building a strong foundation within your nutrition program by learning the basics in the beginner's stage.
- Slowly advance through the nutrition stages and don't be afraid to go back to the stages to build momentum, increase consistency and adherence, and thus reap the results.

Within exercise, you need to remember the following:

- Safety, health, consistency, and adherence will override any magical, overpromised or "next best" exercise program.
- Include REF (Realistic, Enjoyable, and Flexible) in your exercise program for more consistency, adherence, and results.
- Slowly advance through your exercise program by adding volume over your training career, make sure you're doing some sort of progressive overload, and understand there will be peaks and valleys throughout your training journey and that's perfectly okay.

You have all the tools, resources, and talent inside of you. Understand that the time is now to make a change. Make sure to develop a relentless mindset and create a crystal clear vision before anything. If there is any adversity thrown your way, which there will be, reframe your mind and think of it as a blessing in disguise and power through it. Along the way, you must develop sound habits all around in order to establish that foundation; make sure to make this a priority. Consistently executing training and nutrition will lead you to the most important pillar of life, which is your health, and the rest of the pillars will flourish. Now go out become dynamic and live a life worth telling a story about.

The New Era of Fitness Resource Page

Along our fitness journey, we have found many useful resources for our clients and ourselves. We mentioned all of these resources within the chapters of *The New Era of Fitness*. If you want to learn more about overall fitness (exercise, nutrition, mindset, and lifestyle), we hope you'll take some time to check them out.

Our Mentors' Websites

- Layne Norton - PhD Nutritional Sciences, Bodybuilder, Powerlifter, Coach.
  https://www.biolayne.com/

- Lewis Howes - Author, Lifestyle Entrepreneur, and Speaker.
  http://lewishowes.com/

- Tai Lopez - Author, Speaker, Investor, and Entrepreneur.
  http://www.tailopez.com/

- Eric Helms - MS, MPhil, CSCS, USAW L1, Team 3DMJ Coach, PNBA Pro Qualified Bodybuilder, IPF Raw Powerlifter
  http://www.3dmusclejourney.com/

- Chris Record - Internet Marketer, Speaker, and Entrepreneur. www.chrisrecord.com

- Josh Phelan-Life Coach https://fromstrugglecomesstrength.com/sales-page

Books

- *Relentless: From Good to Great to Unstoppable*
  by Tim Grover
  Find out more here:
  www.TheNewEraOfFitness.com/relentless

- *Unbeatable Mind: Forge Resiliency and Mental Toughness to Succeed at an Elite Level* (Third Edition)
  by Mark Devine
  Find out more here:
  www.TheNewEraOfFitness.com/unbeatable

- *H3 Leadership: Be Humble. Stay Hungry. Always Hustle.*
  by Brad Lomenick
  Find out more here:
  www.TheNewEraOfFitness.com/h3

- *The School of Greatness: A Real-World Guide to Living Bigger, Loving Deeper, and Leaving a Legacy*
  by Lewis Howes
  Find out more here:
  www.TheNewEraOfFitness.com/greatness

- *Focus: The Hidden Driver of Excellence*
  by Daniel Goleman
  Find out more here:
  www.TheNewEraOfFitness.com/focus

- *The Muscle and Strength Pyramid Nutrition and The Muscle and Strength Pyramid Training*
  by Eric Helms and Andrea Valdez
  Find out more here:
  www.TheNewEraOfFitness.com/pyramid

- *The Power of Habit: Why We Do What We Do in Life and Business*
  by Charles Duhig
  Find out more here:
  www.TheNewEraOfFitness.com/habit

- *Understanding Nutrition*
  by Ellie Whitney and Sharon Rolfes
  Find out more here:
  www.TheNewEraOfFitness.com/understanding

- *Essentials of Strength Training and Conditioning*
  by Thomas Baechle and Roger Earle
  Find out more here:
  www.TheNewEraOfFitness.com/essentials

- *Practical Programming for Strength Training*
  by Mark Rippetoe and Andy Baker
  Find out more here:
  www.TheNewEraOfFitness.com/practical

- *Science and Practice of Strength Training*
  by Vladimir Zatsiorsky
  Find out more here:
  www.TheNewEraOfFitness.com/science

- *Periodization: Theory and Methodology of Training* (5th edition) by Tudor Bompa and Gregory Haff.
  Find out more here:
  www.TheNewEraOfFitness.com/periodization

About The Authors

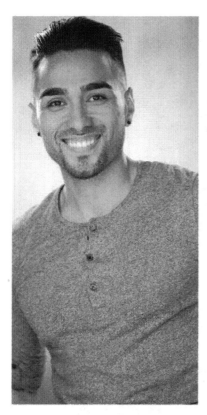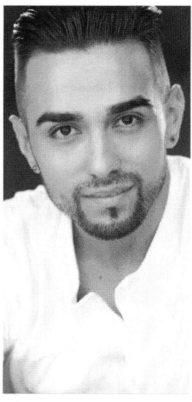

CHRIS and ERIC MARTINEZ, CISSN, CSCS, CPT, BA, are #1 Best Selling Authors and the founders of Dynamic Duo Training. The twin brothers, known as the "Dynamic Duo," have quickly become the leading authorities on health, training, nutrition, and lifestyle in the fitness industry. They provide world class trainings and services with safe, ethical, scientific, and healthy approaches. With a heap of success stories from clients, Chris and Eric have shown time and time again that they know exactly how to get you results. Their online trainings are some of the most talked about in the industry because they get results where other haven't. For more information on the Dynamic Duo's online trainings and to join the DDT community visit www.DynamicDuoTraining.com/special-offer

Other places to find the Dynamic Duo:

- **Dynamic Duo Training** - http://dynamicduotraining.com
- **FaceBook Page** - https://www.facebook.com/dynamicduotraining
- **Twitter** - http://twitter.com/Dynamicduotrain
- **YouTube Channel** - http://www.youtube.com/Dynamicduotraining
- **Instagram** - http://instagram.com/dynamicduotraining
- **Snapchats** - http://dynamicduotraining.com/snap-chat

Made in the USA
San Bernardino, CA
14 October 2016